Pre-Test Study Manual for the

Test of Essential Academic Skills

Reading, Mathematics, Science, and English and Language Usage

Edition 3.0

ATI would like to thank the following individuals for their contributions:

Martin Bartholow, PhD, Shawnee Mission Public Schools

George Chaney, PhD, Ottawa University

Charles George, PhD, North Carolina Central University

Marion F. Gooding, RN, PhD, North Carolina Central University

Janice Van Gorp, MS, Shawnee Mission Public Schools

Jim Hartman, MS, BA, Central Heights High School

Susan Kerr, MA, BA, University of Kansas

Roselyn Laven, MS, Shawnee Mission Public Schools

Mattie E. Moss, EdD, North Carolina Central University

Canda Mueller, PhD(c), Salina Public Schools

James M. Schooler, PhD, North Carolina Central University

Doris E. Wilson, BA, Sampson G. Smith School

Amanda A. Wolkowitz, MS, University of Kansas

Important Notice to the Reader of this Publication

Table of Contents

Section I: Introduction

An Overview

Thank you for purchasing the Test of Essential Academic Skills™ (TEAS™) Pre-Test Study Manual. This book contains instructional material for each of the four subject areas, practice tests and answer keys, and a comprehensive test and answer key.

When creating the TEAS™ Pre-Test Study Manual, the developers had two primary objectives, (1) to design an examination that is voluntary, readily available, and able to be completed in a non-threatening environment, and (2) to develop an instructional module that is closely parallel to the proctored TEAS™ examination.

About the Proctored TEAS™ Examination

The TEAS™ examination was developed to measure basic essential skills in the academic content area domains of Reading, Mathematics, Science, and English and Language Usage. These entry level skills were deemed important for nursing program applicants by a panel of nursing program curriculum experts.

The TEAS™ examination is a 170-item, four-option, multiple-choice examination offered in both paper and pencil and computer-administered format. To prepare in an organized and efficient manner, you should know what to expect from the real examination. Information about the content of the actual examination is given below:

Content Area	Number of Test Items
Reading	40
Mathematics	45
Science	30
English and Language Usage	55
TEAS™ Total	**170**

The Pre-Test Study Manual Section by Section

This study manual is similar to the TEAS™ produced by Assessment Technologies Institute™ (ATI) in that the broad areas of subject matter reflect the sections of the test (Reading, Mathematics, Science, and English and Language Usage). The test questions are multiple choice. You are expected to interpret data, analyze and draw conclusions from data, as well as apply principles and concepts to a variety of situations.

The Reading section of the TEAS™ reviews various styles of reading. The intended purpose for reading and the desired comprehension levels are paired.

The Mathematics section is organized around the major numerical concepts, including whole numbers and integers, fractions and decimals, percents, ratios and proportions, algebra, measurement, and graphs and diagrams. When studying this section it is recommended that you follow the sequence as presented. It is important to understand whole numbers, for example, before moving on to fractions and decimals.

In the Science section, a glossary is provided along with the other instructional material. Knowledge of these basic terms will assist in understanding the material. The material covered in the Science section is far more broad than in the other sections. It reflects both scientific content area knowledge such as Earth Science, General Science, Life Science, Chemistry, and Physics, and multiple aspects of the scientific inquiry process.

The English and Language Usage section emphasizes the rules for the English language and word power achieved through contextual vocabulary. Specific content includes punctuation, grammar, sentence structure, contextual words, and spelling.

Study Suggestions

To prepare for taking the TEAS™, you should review each section of the instructional material, then complete the sample test for each section. As a final check, take the comprehensive examination. The answers to these tests are provided so that you may understand what subject areas may require further study. When taking the practice tests and the comprehensive final, consider simulating actual testing conditions as closely as possible. Create an environment with good lighting and minimal distractions and consider timing yourself on the practice tests.

We strongly urge you to start off by setting up a time frame for completing this study guide. You may start with any of the four subject areas as there is no required sequence for the use of this book. What is recommended is that you set aside specific blocks of time for study. A sample study schedule that might be used is presented below.

SUN	MON	TUE	WED	THU	FRI	SAT
				1 6-8 p.m. Reading	2 11-1 p.m. Reading	3 1-4 p.m. Math
4	5 4-6 p.m. Math	6 9-12 p.m. Math	7 4-6 p.m. Math	8 6-8 p.m. Math	9 11-1 p.m. Life Science	10 1-4 p.m. Life Science
11	12 4-6 p.m. Life Science	13 9-12 p.m. Life Science	14 4-6 p.m. Anatomy and Physiology	15 6-8 p.m. Anatomy and Physiology	16 11-1 p.m. Anatomy and Physiology	17
18	19 4-6 p.m. Chemistry and Physics	20 9-12 p.m. Chemistry and Physics	21 4-6 p.m. Chemistry and Physics	22 6-8 p.m. English	23 11-1 p.m. English	24
25	26 4-6 p.m. English	27 Take Comprehensive Test	28 4-6 p.m. Follow-up Study	29 6-8 p.m. Follow-up Study	30 11-1 p.m. Follow-up Study	31

NOTE: If you would like additional TEAS™ preparatory material, a 100-item online practice examination is available. For more information, please visit www.atitesting.com.

General Guidelines for Test-Taking

1. Carefully read the question to determine the objective of the test item. Put the question in your own words.

2. Identify the stem of the question. This is the main concept that will lead you to the correct answer.

3. Carefully read each of the options. This will help to clarify the objective of the test item.

4. Do not over-generalize. Answer the question from the information provided in the stem only. Do not assume, imagine, etc.

5. Eliminate answers that are definitely wrong or implausible.

6. If you do not know the answer, it is better to guess than to leave the item unanswered.

7. Budget your time carefully to ensure that you have enough time to answer all of the questions in a section.

Section II: Reading

Get Reading Ready

The Reading section of this test preparation and study guide is designed to help you, the test-taker, understand the many facets of reading comprehension and their application to test-taking. It focuses on making you aware of how you have been reading until now and guides in adjusting your reading patterns to help you become a more efficient reader and test taker.

The Reading section first outlines various types of reading and explains how to use each kind. Second, it addresses the types of thinking common to reading comprehension. A third subsection deals with the various types of questions. Finally, there is a reading practice test. It is complete with an answer sheet and answer key. Explanatory notes accompany each of the reading comprehension concepts introduced and/or reviewed.

Prep with a Purpose

Think about it. Would you approach the reading of a bestseller with the same intensity that you would apply to your textbooks? The novel is leisure reading, and the textbook is study reading. Each of these types of reading requires distinctly different reading attitudes and reading rates.

Let's take a look at the six basic types of reading and see how you might apply them as you work toward improving your reading comprehension. Your understanding of these reading differences may improve your performance.

Scanning

Have you ever studied for a test by letting your eyes run quickly over the pages of a chapter in your textbook, pausing only to read the chapter title, section headings, bold face or italicized type, and highlighted words or phrases? If so, you have practiced the technique of scanning. Scanning is sometimes referred to as skimming, which probably explains more graphically what this method of reading entails: It is quick and allows you to skip over insignificant material and go directly to more pertinent information. This is an effective strategy to employ when taking a test. Use it to preview the questions and the multiple-choice options.

Idea Reading

Idea reading is a rapid reading technique wherein you read for essential ideas. Your eyes move with great speed and focus on lengthy phrases. Your brain identifies and records only the most important words in these phrases. With maximum concentration, your eyes will reject all other words. Idea reading is difficult to master, but can provide good reading efficiency. It challenges your ability to understand patterns of the English language, particularly in regard to sentence structure. Idea reading is best applied to comprehension test items that solicit generalization, recognition of subject matter, and the drawing of conclusions. These concepts of reading comprehension are thoroughly discussed in the Comprehension section of this unit.

Exploratory Reading

Exploratory reading is the technique used in situations that require you to recognize and understand main ideas more thoroughly. It requires reading more carefully to enable the reader to relate ideas and associate them with prior knowledge of the topic. Exploratory reading is general content reading that requires that you absorb more detail than you would in scanning or idea reading. This technique is often used in reading materials of greater length, such as literature and long magazine articles.

Study Reading

Study reading occurs when you, the reader, must acquire a maximum understanding of principal ideas and how they relate to one another. It combines scanning and thinking, requires greater concentration than the other techniques, and is accomplished at a slower rate. Material is read in smaller units at any one time. Interruption is anticipated in this type of reading; note taking and breaks are a must with this technique, which is most commonly applied to textbook reading.

Critical Reading

Practicing critical reading will equip you to make judgments about what the author wants you to believe. You will need this technique when reading advertisements and magazine articles, which often contain propaganda. It fosters a consideration of what is fact and what is opinion. When you are engaged in critical reading, you are on alert for propaganda devices such as emotional words, bandwagon, and endorsement, all carefully chosen by the author to persuade you to his or her way of thinking. Critical reading is necessary for determining an author's attitude or tone. These types of test items are reviewed in the Comprehension section.

Analytical Reading

Analytical reading is used with study materials, the content of which may be mathematical theorems, problems, and scientific formulas. It requires deep concentration and a questioning mind. Save this technique for your next math or science exam.

Comprehension

Reading comprehension is simply a matter of being able to think about a passage or text from several different perspectives. Depending on the test questions asked, you will evaluate the text in terms of a particular thought process: determining *subject matter;* finding the *main idea;* making *generalizations;* noting *details;* determining *purpose;* drawing *conclusions;* determining *applications;* identifying *tone and attitude;* understanding *vocabulary;* and identifying *communication techniques.* The table that follows illustrates how this works.

Type of Question	Thought Process
What is the entire passage about?	I'm being asked to identify *subject matter.*
What are the essential points of the passage?	I'm being asked to find the *main idea.* The main idea is the one that is supported by other material or information.
What are the specific facts or opinions used?	I'm being asked to locate *details.*
What does the author want you to do or believe?	I will need to consider the *purpose* of the main idea or generalization here.
What conclusions can be drawn from the generalizations or the details of the passage?	I must look for main ideas stated or implied and the details that support them. From these statements or inferences, I can draw *conclusions.*
How can you apply the conclusions you have made about a passage to new situations not addressed in the passage?	This question asks me to *apply* the conclusions I have drawn and use them to determine new conclusions in situations that share some similarity to those in the passage.
What is the feeling or attitude of the author toward the subject matter of the passage?	I must look for words in this passage that express feelings. I am focusing on the writer's *tone* and *attitude.*
What is the general meaning of a word as used in the passage?	"As used in the passage" is the key phrase in this question. I must consider the words or sentences surrounding this unfamiliar term to determine its meaning. I must be focused on *vocabulary* in context.
What do you notice about the organization of the passage or how are the generalizations related to each other?	How does the author communicate ideas to me? I am looking for *communication techniques.*

Below is a reading passage followed by a series of multiple-choice test items. First, read the questions and the answer choices. See if you can determine the thought process needed to answer each question. Then read the passage and answer the questions. Check your answers using the answer key that follows the questions.

The state is again in financial ruin and it's time to lean on the ever-shrinking pool of smokers. I am always amazed that governors and legislators become so concerned about the health of this despised group whenever large deficits appear. If the legislature were so interested in curing smoking addiction, why not raise the tax to $10 a pack? Based on popular logic, that would certainly be a deterrent.

The latest statistics indicate that obesity is a larger burden on our collective health and insurance costs than smoking. It shouldn't be long before we see the Twinkie tax. We'll need revenue from a new source once all the smokers have died or have been forced to quit.

It would only seem fair that if smokers are forced to bear the fiscal burdens, the smoking bans in government-owned buildings should be lifted so smokers may light up wherever they please. Also, the next time you are in a restaurant, irritated by the cigarette smoke of the person at the table next to you, give him a big "thank you." He may well be responsible for keeping your property taxes stable.

---

1. What is the author's attitude toward the cigarette tax?
    a. humorous
    b. indifferent
    c. disapproving
    d. uneasy

2. Fiscal means:
    a. physical.
    b. refuted.
    c. alleged.
    d. financial.

3. This selection can best be titled:
    a. "Thank a Smoker."
    b. "State Tax Hikes."
    c. "A Smoke-Free State."
    d. "Tax Terror."

4. Legislators appear to be concerned about:
   a. health insurance costs.
   b. property tax.
   c. smoking bans.
   d. the health of smokers.

5. The author uses the word "forced to bear" and "Twinkie tax" to:
   a. add humor to the selection.
   b. dramatize the unfairness of the cigarette tax.
   c. predict future taxes.
   d. discourage smoking.

6. What is the main idea of the passage?
   a. Governors and legislators want to raise cigarette taxes to cover deficits.
   b. Governors and legislators are fighting for smoke-free restaurants.
   c. Smokers should stand up for their rights.
   d. This is about to become a smoke-free state.

7. What attitude does the author recommend we have toward smokers?
   a. concern
   b. gratitude
   c. anger
   d. elation

8. If the cigarette tax was raised to $10 per pack, what effect would this likely have on the smoking population?
   a. The number of people who quit smoking would be significant.
   b. Tobacco companies would go bankrupt.
   c. Fewer teens would smoke.
   d. Smoking would increase.

9. Based on the information in the passage, the reader can assume that smokers are:
   a. ignored by others.
   b. oppressed.
   c. discriminated against.
   d. admirable people.

ANSWER KEY

1. attitude, tone: c
2. vocabulary: d
3. main idea: a
4. detail: d
5. communication techniques: b
6. main idea: a
7. purpose: b
8. application: a
9. conclusion: c

Different Formats of Reading Comprehension Test Items

Paragraphs and Passages

Reading comprehension tests have a distinct format, and test items are usually presented in the form of short paragraphs or, in many instances, longer passages followed by a series of multiple-choice questions. Some test items may appear in the form of a sentence stem to be completed by one of four lettered choices.

> *Example:* *This small, quaint, town is faced with the problem of:*
> *a. mass unemployment.*
> *b. failing lumber mills.*
> *c. air pollution.*
> *d. an AIDS epidemic.*
>
> *Answer:* *c. air pollution*

Other test items may require you to fill in a blank, completing the sentence:

> *Example:* *Passing the budget requires a _____ vote of the organization's financial members.*
> *a. 1/2*
> *b. 3/5*
> *c. 2/3*
> *d. 2/4*
>
> *Answer:* *c. 2/3*

When approaching the short paragraph or passage-reading test item, be certain to apply the techniques reviewed in the Comprehension section. Adjust your reading speed and attitude to skimming mode. Read the question first and then the answer choices. Skim the paragraph for indicators that you can relate to the question and its possible answers. Skimming the paragraph is particularly effective when the answers are short, as in the examples above.

After skimming, remember to read straight through the passage at your usual reading speed. Questions referencing the passage's details may require you to go back to identify more exact information in order to make an appropriate answer choice. Your previewing will help you recall the approximate location of the word(s) or phrase(s) that will supply the answer to the question.

Charts, Maps, Diagrams, and Graphs

Another way of testing reading comprehension is to have test-takers interact with printed images such as charts, diagrams, and graphs. Questions for these test items may require you to interpret information provided by these images. Again, items are presented in a multiple-choice format. It is important to first look for key words in the questions. Try to find information that aligns with the answer choices. This will help you draw conclusions as requested by the question.

Study the chart below and the questions following it. Look for key words in the questions that will tell you what information is needed to answer the questions. Be sure to find information that supports or does not support each of the answer choices. This will help you draw the conclusions as required by some of the questions.

1. If you are planning to spend your August vacation fishing, which week would be the best week to schedule it?
    a. August 24-30
    b. June 3-10
    c. August 17-23
    d. August 3-9

    Note: The key words in the question above are *fishing*, *best*, *week,* and *August*. This question is actually asking you to conclude when is the best time for the best fishing. You are looking for a block of time in *August* (the calendar is for the month of August only) that amounts to a calendar week. "Best" fishing is represented by the symbol of all black or colored-in fish. Look for the calendar week which has the most days with the "best fishing" symbol. That would be August 17-23. The answer would be *c*.

2. If you went fishing August 14-21, on which day would you be LEAST likely to bring home some fish?
    a. 14th
    b. 16th
    c. 18th
    d. 21st

    Note: The key words in this question are *day* and *least*. The term *least* in this question translates to *poorest*. Consult the chart for a symbol for "poor" fishing. The unfilled-in outline of a fish represents poor fishing. This symbol appears on August 14th. The answer would be *a*.

Following Directions

Still another kind of reading comprehension test item takes you through a set of **step-by-step** directions. It is imperative that you perform each step accurately in the sequence it is given. The final step will bring you to a solution or result that is the same as one of the choices for an answer. Here's how:

Example: *Complete the following steps in the order they appear. Then answer the question that follows.*

1. *Draw a square.*
2. *Draw a triangle on the top of the square whose base shares the topside of the square.*
3. *Draw a triangle whose base shares the right side of the square.*
4. *Repeat number 3 for the left side of the square.*
5. *Place a bold dot in the middle of the square.*
6. *Repeat step 2 for the bottom of the square.*

Which figure is most like your drawing?

a.
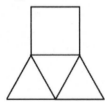

b.
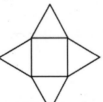

c.
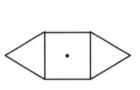

d.
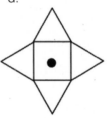

Note: If you drew the figure step by step, it should resemble **d**. The directions required that you draw one square and four triangles. That would eliminate figure **a** and figure **c**. You were also instructed to place a bold dot in the center of the square. Figure **b** does not have a dot. Figure **d** has four triangles, all of which have bases that share sides with the square. It also has a pronounced dot in the center of the square.

Test-Taking Strategies Review

Let's put what you have practiced to use. The practice test that follows encompasses many of the types of comprehension questions reviewed in this unit. It requires you to utilize all of the test-taking strategies outlined. In preparing to take the practice test or an actual standardized reading exam, keep in mind some basic "rules of thumb."

- Skim questions pertaining to all reading paragraphs or passages and the choices provided for answers.

- Be aware of words in each passage that signal the details of who, what, when, why, and how. Proper nouns and/or prepositional phrases beginning with at, on, near, by, above, etc. should alert you to details.

- Go back and read the passage at regular speed to find specific information before answering questions.

- If you encounter an unfamiliar word, examine the words surrounding the unknown term that could help you determine its meaning. If the test question asks for the meaning of a word, take your time to avoid making careless mistakes. For example, when looking for synonyms, avoid answer choices that look overly similar to the target word, such as *simile* and *smile*. Also, make certain that the word you choose for an answer is the same part of speech as the word in question; for instance, the adverb *slowly* could not be a synonym for the verb *retard*.

- When the question asks you to select a word or phrase to complete a sentence, read the question at least twice. Then read the question again, each time completing the sentence with one of the answer choices. This process takes only seconds and will help you determine the most appropriate answer.

- If the test item addresses the order of events, pay attention to words that indicate sequence (first, second, before, after, later, next, then).

- Remember that there is only one correct answer; the other answer choices are distracters and are designed to force you to employ an effective thought process to complete the answer.

Test Information

The reading practice test you are about to take is multiple choice with only one correct answer per question. The test is comprised of a variety of short paragraphs, passages, charts, or diagrams. Photocopy the answer sheet on this page to record your choices. Read each test item and circle your answer on the answer sheet. When you have completed the practice test, you may check your answers with those listed on the answer key that follows the Reading Practice Test.

Reading Practice Test
Answer Sheet

Sample Test Items

1. a   b   **c**   d
2. **a**   b   c   d

1.	a	b	c	d	26.	a	b	c	d
2.	a	b	c	d	27.	a	b	c	d
3.	a	b	c	d	28.	a	b	c	d
4.	a	b	c	d	29.	a	b	c	d
5.	a	b	c	d	30.	a	b	c	d
6.	a	b	c	d	31.	a	b	c	d
7.	a	b	c	d	32.	a	b	c	d
8.	a	b	c	d	33.	a	b	c	d
9.	a	b	c	d	34.	a	b	c	d
10.	a	b	c	d	35.	a	b	c	d
11.	a	b	c	d	36.	a	b	c	d
12.	a	b	c	d	37.	a	b	c	d
13.	a	b	c	d	38.	a	b	c	d
14.	a	b	c	d	39.	a	b	c	d
15.	a	b	c	d	40.	a	b	c	d
16.	a	b	c	d	41.	a	b	c	d
17.	a	b	c	d	42.	a	b	c	d
18.	a	b	c	d	43.	a	b	c	d
19.	a	b	c	d	44.	a	b	c	d
20.	a	b	c	d	45.	a	b	c	d
21.	a	b	c	d	46.	a	b	c	d
22.	a	b	c	d	47.	a	b	c	d
23.	a	b	c	d	48.	a	b	c	d
24.	a	b	c	d	49.	a	b	c	d
25.	a	b	c	d	50.	a	b	c	d

Sample Questions

Read each sample question below and mark your answer choice on the answer sheet in the space provided for "sample questions." These sample test items are not to be scored.

1. Kevin needs to review the description of flower parts for a test. To find out where this information is located in his biology textbook, he should look in the:
    a.   table of contents.
    b.   appendix.
    c.   index.
    d.   glossary.

2. Which information is not found on a driver's license?
    a.   place of employment
    b.   home address
    c.   age
    d.   color of eyes

Reading Practice Test

Reading Test

The diagram below is a circle that has been divided into eight parts. Each part is adjacent to two other parts. In other words, each part shares common lines with two other parts. Each section of the circle can be named using the letters that appear within it. For example: JSW means S is positioned between J and W.

It can be said that JSW is true for this diagram because S is between J and W and shares common lines with J and W.

1. Which of the following statements is also true for this diagram?
    a.   WOB
    b.   STM
    c.   BLJ
    d.   OML

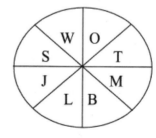

2. What is a synonym for <u>adjacent</u>?
    a.   adjoining
    b.   adherent
    c.   infinite
    d.   adjutant

Read the paragraph below and answer questions 3 through 5.

Freshwater habitats are distinct from marine and land habitats. Freshwater habitats vary greatly because they include ponds, lakes, bogs, rivers, streams, creeks, marshes, and swamps. All of these make up a very limited area of the earth's surface. Lakes cover only 1.8 percent, and streams and rivers combined make up only 0.3 percent of the total surface area of the earth. Considering this, it is amazing to find out how much plant life these freshwater habitats provide. Freshwater habitats produce many times the plant materials in grasslands and even in farmers' fields. These food products are used by animals within the freshwater habitat, but other species that live in surrounding habitats also depend on food and water within the freshwater habitats. In addition, a large amount of organic and inorganic material continuously enters bodies of freshwater from communities on the land nearby. These habitats are not only constantly changing, but they are also moving. Species living in freshwater habitats must be able to swim against currents or attach themselves in some way in order to escape being swept away. All of these make the freshwater habitat and the animals that live within them unique.

3. The purpose of this passage is to:
    a. entertain.
    b. express a feeling.
    c. persuade.
    d. inform.

4. The main thought here is that freshwater habitats:
    a. have a connection to other habitats.
    b. differ greatly from marine and land habitats.
    c. can support many kinds of organisms.
    d. cover about 2.1% of the earth's surface.

5. According to the passage, marshes and swamps are categorized as:
    a. freshwater habitats.
    b. marine habitats.
    c. land habitats.
    d. streams.

Use the information on the weather chart to answer questions 6 through 8.

NATION

	TODAY			TOMORROW		
	HI	LO	W	HI	LO	W
Albuquerque	94	74	s	94	62	s
Atlanta	82	62	s	83	64	c
Baltimore	78	60	t	80	62	t
Biloxi, MS	91	71	s	86	72	pc
Boise	92	60	s	92	58	s
Boston	56	51	r	64	57	t
Branson, MO	83	58	pc	79	59	pc
Buffalo	65	53	r	63	53	sh
Charleston, SC	88	64	s	88	68	s
Chicago	71	52	s	88	68	s
Cleveland	66	556	sh	66	52	sh
Dallas	88	68	s	84	68	t
Denver	80	52	t	83	58	t
Detroit	68	55	sh	66	52	sh
Fairbanks	76	48	s	75	50	s
Hartford	64	52	r	68	56	t
Honolulu	87	74	pc	87	74	s
Houston	92	72	s	90	73	c
Kansas City	82	56	pc	80	61	sh
Las Vegas	104	76	s	104	76	s
Los Angeles	71	61	pc	71	61	pc
Miami	86	74	t	88	74	sh
Milwaukee	69	54	pc	69	54	pc
Minneapolis	72	51	p	75	56	t
New Orleans	90	69	s	85	71	pc
New York	66	58	sh	72	58	t
Norfolk	84	64	t	84	66	pc
Omaha	83	55	pc	79	60	s
Orlando	92	71	t	92	71	pc
Philadelphia	76	58	t	76	60	t
Phoenix	109	82	s	109	82	s
Seattle	72	52	s	70	54	pc
Tampa	90	75	pc	90	76	s
Washington, DC	78	62	t	80	62	t
Wichita	82	56	c	80	61	t
Wilmington, DE	76	58	t	79	60	t

pc	partly cloudy
r	rain
t	thunderstorm
s	sunny
sh	showers

6. According to the nation's weather chart, what cities will be experiencing showers today?
   a. Seattle, New York and Dallas
   b. Boston, Buffalo and Fairbanks
   c. Cleveland, Dallas and Miami
   d. New York, Detroit and Cleveland

7. Which city cannot look forward to the exact same temperatures for two days in succession?
   a. Las Vegas
   b. Los Angeles
   c. Philadelphia
   d. Honolulu

8. Which major league baseball team is most likely to have its home game called off today due to inclement weather?
   a. Baltimore Orioles
   b. Kansas City Royals
   c. Milwaukee Brewers
   d. Atlanta Braves

Use the information from the Drug label to answer questions 9 and 10.

9. People with which of the following medical conditions should avoid using this medicine?
   a. flu
   b. arthritis
   c. diabetes
   d. asthma

10. This medication is used to treat::
    a. glaucoma.
    b. bronchitis.
    c. runny nose.
    d. enlarged prostate.

SEALED IN BLISTER UNIT FOR YOUR PROTECTION

Drug Facts

Active ingredient (in each tablet)	Purpose
Chlorpheniramine maleate 4 mg...Antihistamine	

Uses ■ temporarily relieves these symptoms of hay fever or other upper respiratory allergies:
■ runny nose ■ sneezing ■ itchy nose or throat ■ itchy, watery eyes

Warnings

Ask a doctor before use if you have ■ glaucoma ■ trouble urinating due to an enlarged prostate gland
■ a breathing problem such as emphysema or chronic bronchitis

Ask a doctor or pharmacist before use if you are taking sedatives or tranquilizers

When using this product ■ alcohol, sedatives and tranquilizers may increase drowsiness
■ drowsiness may occur ■ avoid alcoholic drinks ■ excitability may occur, especially in children
■ be careful when driving a motor vehicle or operating machinery

If pregnant or breast-feeding, ask a health professional before use.
Keep out of reach of children. In case of overdose, get medical help or contact a Poison
Control Center right away.

Directions ■ take every 4 to 6 hours, not more than 6 doses in 24 hours

adults and children 12 years and over	1 tablet (4 mg)
children 6 to under 12 years	1/2 tablet (2 mg)
children under 6 years	ask a doctor

Other information ■ store at room temperature ■ protect from moisture

Inactive ingredients corn starch, D&C yellow no. 10, lactose, magnesium stearate

Study the map and answer questions 11 through 13.

11. Which of the following statements is true?
    a. Meadow View Plaza is directly accessible from Rt. 287.
    b. Route 22 and 95 do not merge in the vicinity of Newark Airport.
    c. Cranford is north of Iselin.
    d. Meadow View Plaza is located in Basking Ridge.

12. The Garden State Parkway runs:
    a. east and west.
    b. north and south.
    c. parallel to Rt. 22.
    d. into Rt. 21.

13. Traveling north from Woodbridge on 95, which town will you arrive at first?
    a. Secaucus
    b. Union
    c. Edison
    d. Elizabeth

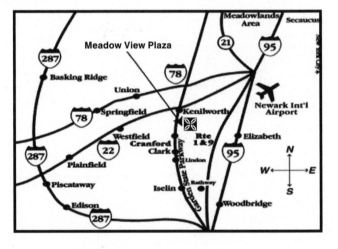

Use the ad below to answer questions 14 through 16.

ATHLETIC DIRECTOR

Hanover Public Schools invites outstanding educators to apply for the position of Athletic Director. The Athletic Director will have responsibility to develop and supervise the interscholastic athletic program.

We are seeking an innovative, dynamic and results-oriented leader with a proven record of accomplishment.

Qualifications:

• Master's degree in Physical Education or Athletic Administration preferred
• Eligible for a New Jersey Supervisor Certificate
• Five years of successful experience as a teacher and coach of an interscholastic athletic team
• Record of successful experience in supervision and evaluation
• Ability to build productive and collaborative relationships with staff, students and parents
• Experience in data analysis, preparing budgets

Highly competitive salary and fringe benefit package. Position effective immediately.

Send letter of interest, resume and copy of certificate by June 28, 2002 to:

Ms. Ana Castillo
Director of Human Resources
Hanover Public Schools
235 Valley Way, Hanover, NJ 07352
www.hanover.k12.nj.us

Hanover values diversity. An Equal Opportunity Employer/Affirmative Action Employer.

14. According to the advertisement, what statement is true?
    a. Ms. Ana Castillo is the current athletic director.
    b. A Master's Degree in Athletic Administration is not a necessary qualification.
    c. The position will become available on June 28, 2002.
    d. No previous experience is required.

15. The ad was placed by an employer who is:
    a. looking for a physical education teacher.
    b. not willing to negotiate salary.
    c. planning to eliminate the interview process.
    d. considering candidates of all races, creeds, and genders for the posted position.

16. Eligible means the same as:
    a. edible.
    b. legal.
    c. possible.
    d. qualified.

Use the television programming guide below to answer questions 17 through 19.

Saturday Morning and Early Afternoon

AM	7:00	7:30	8:00	8:30	9:00	9:30	10:00	10:30	11:00	11:30	12:00	12:30
2/3	Bob Build	Dora...	Blue's	Little Bill	The Saturday Early Show Messages, online safety. (cc)				Franklin	Oswald	Paid Prog.	Paid Prog.
4/10	Today Sarah Brightman performs. (cc)			News (cc)		City /Guys	Skate	NBA	City Guys	About Us	Just Deal	Gold U.S. Open.
9	Paid Prog.	Key/David	Paid Prog.	Paid Prog.	Paid Prog.	Paid Prog.	Paid Prog.	Paid Prog.	Paid Prog.	In House	Paid Prog.	Paid Prog.
11	Time	S. Holmes	Rescue	Static Shk.	J. Chan	Powerpuff	Pokemon	Yu-Gi-Oh!	X-Men	Phantom	City Guys	City Guys
N12	Bus.	Pet Stop	Fast Tr'k	NJ	Health	Stage	Jersey's Talking		TBA	Bus.	Fast Tr'k	Health
12	Suze Orman: The Road to Wealth Financial advice.				Witness to Hope Historic stills and film explore the personal life of Pope John Paul II.					Suze Orman: The Road to Wealth Financial advice.		
13	Defense	Wash.	Ruk.	Trenton	Think	On One	Kno.	Religion	T. Brown	Contrary	Mind	Caucus
17	Tama	Heavy ...	Rescue	Static	J. Chan	'puff	Pokem'n	Yu-Gi	X-Men	Phantom	Wayans	Wayans
21	One Stroke Painting With Donna Dewberry			The Wrinkle Cure With Dr. Nicholas Perricone					Ten Secrets for Success and Inner Peace		Spiritual Solution	
29	Pets	Adven.	Woody	Rangers	Galidor	Digimon	Mdbt.	Digimon	Trans	Knights	Rescue	TWIB
PAX 31	Paid	Paid	Paid	Root's	Paid	Paid	Paid	Paid	Paid	Paid	Paid	Paid
41	Copa Mundial 2002				Planeta U (cc) (TVY)				Super Sabado Sensacional			
47	Tree	Agua V's	Melliza	Bizbirlje	NICO	Toon	Mi Terra		Frente	Notices	Buena O's	

17. What channels feature two-hour blocks of programming on Saturday mornings?
    a. Channels 17 and 47.
    b. Channels 3, 12, and 21.
    c. Channels 4, 9, and 10.
    d. Channels N12 and 41.

18. Which channel has programming that has not yet been announced?
    a. N12 at 11:00 a.m.
    b. Channel 29 at 10:30 a.m.
    c. Channel 13 at 7:00 a.m.
    d. N12 at 9:00 a.m.

19. Which of the following statements is true?
    a. "Pokemon" airs at 10:30 p.m.
    b. PAX 31 is mostly free programming.
    c. "One Stroke Painting with Donna Dewberry" is a 1½ hour show
    d. "Rescue" airs at 9:00 a.m.

Answer the following questions.

20. Which word means the same as infidelity?
    a. unfaithfulness
    b. infinity
    c. infamy
    d. uniformity

21. A recipe lists the following ingredients: sugar, salt, flour, milk, butter, eggs. Step 1 of the directions requires that you mix the dry ingredients in a bowl. Which ingredients would you mix?
    a. eggs, sugar, flour, salt
    b. sugar, salt, flour
    c. butter, baking powder, milk, salt
    d. flour, salt, sugar, milk

Read the following passage and answer questions 22 through 24.

I hear the whistle of the locomotive in the woods... Whew! Whew! Whew! How is real estate here in the swamp and wilderness?

–Ralph Waldo Emerson, 1842

WHICH BRINGS US TO GREATER Atlanta, 1999. Once a wilderness, it's now a 13-county eruption, one that has been called the fastest-spreading human settlement in history. Already more than 110 miles across, up from just 65 in 1990, it consumes an additional 500 acres of field and farmland every week. What it leaves behind is tract houses, access roads, strip malls, off ramps, industrial parks and billboards advertising more tract houses where the peach trees used to be. Car exhaust is such a problem that Washington is withholding new highway funding until the region complies with federal clean-air standards. On a bad traffic day–basically any weekday with a morning and evening in it–you can review whole years of your life in the time it takes to get from Blockbuster to Fuddruckers.

"We can't go on like this," says Georgia Governor Roy Barnes, a "smart growth" Democrat who was elected last year. Barnes has proposed a regional transportation authority that can block local plans for the new roads that encourage development. But dumb growth is not confined to Atlanta. Half a century after America loaded the car and fled to the suburbs, these boundless, slapdash places are making people

22. The best statement of the main idea of this passage is:
   a. Atlanta's growth is consuming farm acreage.
   b. Atlanta has been the inspiration for other cities' rapid growth.
   c. rapid growth and over development of a city is neither environmentally sound nor conducive to comfortable living.
   d. politicians have encouraged Atlanta's hasty growth as a vote-getting tactic.

23. The author strongly implies that:
   a. sprawling cities are desirable environments.
   b. plans for Atlanta's growth have not been considerate of environmental issues.
   c. he is in favor of the "sprawling city" concept.
   d. tract homes provide affordable residential areas.

24. The phrase "13-county eruption" suggests:
   a. thoughtless growth.
   b. a positive direction for Atlanta.
   c. a literal explosion has taken place.
   d. devastation of a rural community.

Read the following passage and answer questions 25 through 27.

> The chemical carcinogenesis theory was first advanced in 1761 by Dr. John Hill, an English physician who noted unusual tumors of the nose in heavy snuff users and suggested that tobacco had produced these cancers. In 1775, a London surgeon, Sir Percivall Pott, made a similar observation, noting that men who had been chimney sweeps exhibited frequent cancer of the scrotum, and suggested that soot and tars might be responsible. (British chimney sweeps washed themselves infrequently and always seemed covered with soot; chimney sweeps on the continent, however, who washed daily, had much less of this scrotal cancer.) These and many other observations led to the hypothesis that cancer results from the action of chemicals on the body.

25. This paragraph focuses on:
    a. chemicals that cause cancer.
    b. the history and background of the carcinogenesis theory.
    c. cleanliness and hygiene as preventive measures in the fight against cancer.
    d. Dr. John Hill's contribution to cancer research.

26. Early observations suggest that:
    a. certain chemicals, when applied to or brought in contact with the body, act as carcinogens.
    b. soot and tars cause lung cancer.
    c. tumors of the nose are usually malignant.
    d. snuff was a major cause of cancer.

27. Both Dr. John Hill and Sir Percivall Pott were:
    a. surgeons.
    b. English.
    c. cancer victims.
    d. involved in chemical research.

Answer questions 28 and 29 based on the advertisement below.

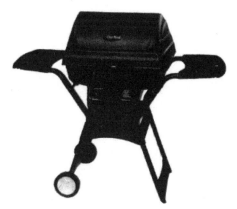

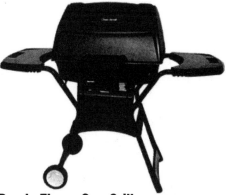

Char-Broil Ready Flame Gas Grill
- 35,000 BTU
- 340 sq. in cooking area
- Push button ignition
- Porcelain cooking grid
- Plastic side shelves with tool hanger
- LP tank included

$139

Ready Flame Gas Grill
- 40,000 BTU ✔
- 780 sq. in total cooking area ✔
- Push button ignition
- Porcelain cooking grid
- Plastic side shelves with tool hanger
- Swing-away warming rack ✔
- LP tank included

$169

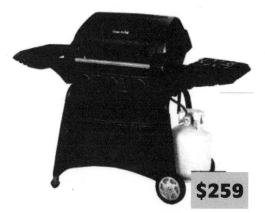

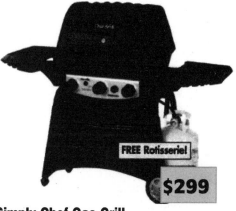

$259

FREE Rotisserie!

$299

Simply Chef Gas Grill/Smoker with Sideburner
- 35,000 BTU
- 585 sq. in. total cooking surface
- Fast start electronic ignition
- 3 stainless steel Readylight burners
- 179 sq. in. AdjustaBlaza warming rack
- Includes LP tank

Simply Chef Gas Grill
- 36,000 BTU with an 11,000 BTU rotisserie
- 585 sq. in. total cooking area
- Fast start electronic ignition
- Porcelain cast-iron grates and grid
- Three stainless steel burners and Readylight
- Includes LP tank

28. The differences between the $139 grill and the $169 grill are the:
    a. cooking area, swing-away warming rack, and the BTUs.
    b. free griddle, rotisserie, and push button ignition.
    c. BTUs, plastic side shelves, and cooking area.
    d. LP tank and porcelain cooking grill.

29. Which grill has the larger cooking surface and push-button ignition as well?
    a. $139 grill
    b. $169 grill
    c. $259 grill
    d. $299 grill

Read the following passage and answer questions 30 through 32.

The 2,315-mile Missouri River tops this year's list of the "10 Most Endangered Rivers in North America," compiled annually by the conservation group American Rivers. The "Big Muddy" has been dammed, channeled, and diked to the point that one-fifth of the species native to the river and its floodplain are now classified as endangered, threatened, or of special concern, according to American Rivers. The other nine rivers on the list are New York's Upper Hudson, Washington's White Salmon, California's San Joaquin, Wisconsin's Wolf River, Arizona's Pinto Creek and Potomac, Ohio's Mill Creek, the Lower Colorado and the Tennessee River.

30. The "Big Muddy" is a reference to what river?
    a. White Salmon
    b. Lower Colorado
    c. Missouri
    d. San Joaquin

31. It may be concluded that:
    a. bodies of water with "creek" in their names are not rivers.
    b. Wolf River is located in Washington, DC.
    c. the damming, diking, and channeling of a river is detrimental to the organisms that inhabit it.
    d. the rivers of North America have been found to be more endangered than those of South America.

32. A conservation group organizes for the principal purpose of:
    a. collecting data.
    b. saving rain forests.
    c. channeling rivers.
    d. preserving nature.

Read the following passage and answer questions 33 through 35.

And so we are gathered here today — you, the eager members of the class of 2002, and we, your family members, who will sit on these hard folding chairs until every last eager one of you has picked up a diploma, at which point we will feel as though the entire River Dance troupe has been stomping on our buttocks.

Because, gosh, there sure are a lot of you in the class of 2002! We in the audience are wondering if there is anybody in North America, besides us, who is not graduating today. And although we know this is very exciting for you, the class of 2002, we are fighting to stay awake.

We have already engaged in the traditional time-passing activities of commencement audiences, such as trying to remember the names of all Seven Dwarfs and looking through the commencement program for comical graduate names. We have nudged the person sitting next to us and pointed to names like Konrad A. Klamsucker Jr. and Vorbama Frepitude, and that has given us brief moments of happiness.

But we can do that only for so long, class of 2002, and now we are feeling the despair that comes over members of a commencement audience when they realize that 40 minutes have passed, and the dean is just now starting to hand out diplomas to people whose last names start with D, and the last name of the one graduate we actually came to see starts with W.

We've decided that, if we ever have another child threatening to graduate from college, we're going to have that child's name legally changed to Aaron A. Aardvark. Yes, the other families in the audience will make fun of it. But their laughter will turn to bitter envy when our child gets his diploma first, and we get up off these folding chairs and head for a restaurant! Ha ha!

We also think it would be nice if commencement programs had interesting articles for the audience to read, or even short works of fiction.

33. The author's attitude toward graduation ceremonies is:
    a. indifferent.
    b. humorous.
    c. angry.
    d. morbid.

34. The phrase "as though the entire River Dance troupe has been stomping on our buttocks" is an example of:
    a. onomatopoeia.
    b. simile.
    c. hyperbole.
    d. metaphor.

35. The author finds graduation exercises:
    a. boring.
    b. engaging.
    c. exhilarating.
    d. sentimental.

Read the passage below and review the THR chart that follows to answer questions 36 through 38.

Target heart rate (THR) is a common way to determine how hard you should exercise during endurance activities. It indicates how fast the average person's heart should beat during endurance sessions. It's not always the best way for older adults to decide how hard to exercise, though, because many have long-standing medical conditions or take medications that change their heart rates. However, exercisers who are in basically good health and who like taking a "scientific" approach to their endurance activities may find the THR method useful. Others should check with a doctor first.

For those of you who can use THR, the chart in the right-hand column shows an estimate of how fast you should try to make your heart beat, once you have gradually worked your way up to it.

36. THR is:
   a. a method of exercising.
   b. a stress test.
   c. an approach to improving your physical exercise regimen.
   d. a measurement of how fast the average person should make his/her heart beat while engaging in endurance sessions.

Age	Desired Range for Heart During Endurance Exercise (beats per minute)
20	140-170
30	132-162
40	126-153
50	119-145
60	112-136
70	105-128
80	98-119
90	91-111

37. The THR method would NOT be recommended for adults:
   a. with chronic illnesses.
   b. who jog.
   c. who are overweight.
   d. with vision problems.

38. It may be concluded that the THR for your son would be:
   a. lower than yours.
   b. in the same range as yours.
   c. higher than yours.
   d. more irregular than yours.

Answer the following questions.

39. How many syllables are in the word incomprehensible?
   a. three
   b. four
   c. six
   d. seven

40. The guide words at the top of the dictionary page are dextral and diamond. Which word would be an entry on this page?
   a. diamagnetic
   b. dexterity
   c. devilry
   d. dewdrop

Review the chart below and answer questions 41 through 44.

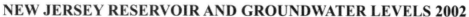

NEW JERSEY RESERVOIR AND GROUNDWATER LEVELS 2002

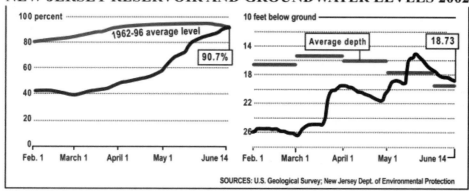

SOURCES: U.S. Geological Survey; New Jersey Dept. of Environmental Protection

41. Measurements of reservoir and groundwater levels on the chart above show that the precipitation:
    a. has increased from March to June.
    b. has been more than the average for 1962-1996.
    c. has not been sufficient to end the drought emergency.
    d. was plentiful in January.

42. During which month were reservoir levels at their lowest?
    a. February
    b. March
    c. April
    d. June

43. Reservoir levels have risen ___ percent during a period from March to June.
    a. 40%
    b. 50%
    c. 70%
    d. 80%

44. The average depth of groundwater levels is:
    a. 16.2 feet.
    b. 18.73 feet.
    c. 23.2 feet.
    d. 31.7 feet.

Answer the following questions.

45.   Zewei appeared <u>rapturous</u> when he received a C in chemistry; his mother, on the contrary, looked displeased. <u>Rapturous</u> means:
   a.   rattled.
   b.   dismayed.
   c.   ecstatic.
   d.   ravenous.

46.   Mrs. Crawford is a <u>gregarious</u> individual who enjoys joining groups and interacting with people. <u>Gregarious</u> means:
   a.   fraternizing.
   b.   introverted.
   c.   gregarine.
   d.   reclusive.

Complete the following in the exact sequence given, then answer question 47.

---

   1.   Draw a circle.
   2.   Draw a square inside the circle.
   3.   Draw a line diagonally from the top left corner of the square to the bottom right corner of the square.
   4.   Draw a line diagonally from the top right corner of the square to the bottom left corner of the square.

---

47.   Which figure is most like your drawing?
   a.   c.

   b.   d.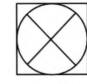

Answer the following questions.

48. You are interested in placing an ad in the newspaper to sell your car. To which department of the newspaper should you e-mail the information?
   a. Editorial
   b. Business
   c. Local News
   d. Classified

49. Which of these is most appropriate to use as personal identification?
   a. insurance certificate
   b. ATM card
   c. marriage certificate
   d. driver's license

50. To locate the address and phone number of a business to assist you with furnishing your new home, you should look in the phone book under:
   a. "Interiors."
   b. "Landscaping."
   c. "Curtains and Draperies."
   d. "Dinettes."

END OF THE TEST

Reading Practice Test Answer Key

1.   c   BLJ is the only answer with adjacent lines.

2.   a   <u>Adjacent</u> means to be "next to one another" or "adjoining."

3.   d   The paragraph was written to inform its readers about freshwater habitats.

4.   b   The only correct answer for the main thought is freshwater habitats differ from marine and land habitats.

5.   a   In the second sentence of the paragraph, marshes and swamps are categorized as freshwater habitats.

6.   d   Under the nation's "today" weather chart, New York, Detroit, and Cleveland are the only cities with sh(showers).

7.   c   Philadelphia is the only city listed with differing low temperatures on two successive days.

8.   a   Baseball is played unless there is a thunderstorm. The only city expecting a thunderstorm is Baltimore.

9.   d   None of the answers are listed under the warnings except for asthma, which is a breathing problem.

10.   c   Only "runny nose" is listed under the uses section of the medication.

11.   c   Looking at the map, Cranford is north of Iselin. The other choices are false.

12.   b   The Garden State Parkway runs up and down, which is north and south.

13.   d   According to the map, the next town going north from Woodbridge on 95 is Elizabeth.

14.   b   Ms. Ana Castillo is the Director of Human Resources. The position does not state when the position comes available. Under qualifications, the ad states that the Master's degree is preferred, not required.

15.   d   The ad states "Hanover values diversity and is an equal opportunity employer/affirmative action employer."

16.   d   <u>Eligible</u> means "to be qualified for the job."

17.   b   The only channels that have two-hour blocks of programming are channels 3, 12, and 21.

18.   a   The letters TBA are on channel N12 at 11:00 a.m. They stand for "to be announced." The other choices list specific programs.

19.   c   "Pokemon" airs at 10:00 a.m., not 10:30 p.m. PAX 31 is mostly paid programming. "One Stroke Painting with Donna Dewberry" is a 1 ½ hour show (from 7:00 – 8:30 a.m.) and is the one correct choice.

20.   a   "Unfaithfulness" is the meaning of <u>infidelity</u>.

21.   b   B is the only choice with all dry ingredients.

22.   c   The main idea is that there is rapid growth and over-development of Atlanta and that it is not a positive move.

23.   b   The only correct answer is b because the other three responses look at the growth in a positive way.

24.	a	"Thoughtless growth" expresses the author's opinion of Atlanta's growth and is echoed in the words "dumb growth" in the second paragraph.
25.	b	The main idea of this paragraph is the background of the carcinogenesis theory, not specific facts about cancer.
26.	a	The only correct answer is a; the other choices are too narrow or not proven facts.
27.	b	The correct answer is English. Both men were not surgeons or involved in chemical research. There is nothing in the paragraph that states they were cancer victims.
28.	a	The differences between the $139 grill and the $169 grill are the cooking area (340 square inches versus 780 square inches), the swing-away warming rack (only offered on the $169 grill), and the BTUs (35,000 BTUs versus 40,000 BTUs).
29.	b	The only grill with the largest cooking surface and push-button ignition is the $169 grill.
30.	c	The passage is about endangered rivers in North America. It starts by mentioning the Missouri River and continues to refer to it as the "Big Muddy."
31.	c	The passage explains the impact on the organisms that live there. There is no information about the difference between a creek and a river. Wolf River is located in Wisconsin. There is no information about rivers of South America.
32.	d	The purpose of a conservation group is to preserve nature and not let it become endangered.
33.	b	The author shows humor in his speech by exaggerating and making fun of graduation ceremonies.
34.	b	A simile compares two unlike things using the word like or as.
35.	a	The author finds graduation exercises boring because he tries to make suggestions about how it could be more interesting.
36.	d	THR is a measurement of how fast the average person should make his/her heart beat while engaging in endurance sessions. It is not a method of exercise or a stress test.
37.	a	THR would only be used in exercise during endurance activities, which would not be appropriate for people with chronic illnesses.
38.	c	According to the chart, the younger you are, the higher your THR, so your son's THR would be higher than yours.
39.	c	Syllabication (breaking the word into smaller sound/syllable units as you say it) and the dictionary entry indicate that the word has six syllables.
40.	a	"Diamagnetic" comes after dextral and before diamond in the dictionary.
41.	a	The bold line in the left-hand chart shows an increase from March to June.
42.	b	The chart shows the lowest reservoir levels in March.
43.	b	The reservoir levels have risen from approximately 39% to 90.7%, or around 50%.
44.	a	The average depth of the groundwater can only be 16.2 feet because the average is the measurements added together and then divided by 5.
45.	c	Rapturous means "ecstatic" or "delighted," which is answer c. Ecstatic would be the antonym of "displeased."

46. a   <u>Gregarious</u> means "fraternizing" or "enjoying the interactions of a group of people."

47. c   Figure c contains a square inside a circle and no vertical line.

48. d   If you wanted to sell a car, you would place an ad in the advertising section known as the classifieds.

49. d   A driver's license is a valid form of identification because it has your photograph and identifying information.

50. a   For a general number to furnish your house, you would look under "Interiors." Option b refers to the outdoors, and c and d are too specific.

Section III: Mathematics

This mathematics study guide is designed to prepare you for the TEAS™ mathematics examination. This module will provide you with a review of basic concepts in mathematics. The topics covered in this module are numbers, operations, percents, ratios, proportions, algebra, measurements, graphs, and diagrams. Basic concepts pertaining to each of these topics will be discussed and illustrative problems will be solved. Practice problems follow the topics discussed. A practice test related to the covered topics is also provided. This module includes solutions for all practice problems and practice test questions. You should try finding the solutions yourself before looking at the solutions provided. Solutions for practice problems follow presentations on each topic.

Numbers

Real Numbers

The **real number system** is used in everyday mathematics. There are **subsets** to this system that will be discussed in further detail. The set of real numbers includes the subsets of the counting numbers, whole numbers, integers, rational, and irrational numbers. The following diagrams show how these number types are related.

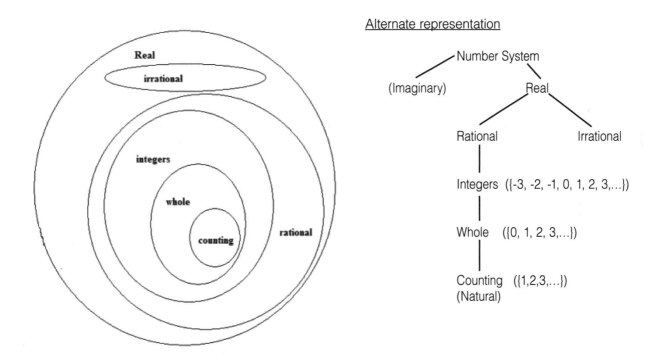

The **counting** numbers (also referred to as the natural numbers or positive integers) are defined as the set {1,2,3,4,...}.

The set of **whole** numbers is the set of counting numbers and 0. In the notation on the previous page, the whole numbers are defined as the set {0,1,2,3...}.

The set of **integers** includes the set of whole numbers and the set of negative counting numbers. A negative counting number is a counting number preceded by a negative sign, (-). That is, negative 3 is written as -3. The set of integers is written as {..., -3,-2,-1,0,1,2,3,...}

Note that each set so far has been composed of non-fraction numbers. Fractions, repeating decimals, and finite decimals, along with the set of integers, compose the set of **rational** numbers. A finite decimal is one that stops, such as 0.25. A repeating decimal is one like 0.333... or 0.167167167... where the 3 and 167 respectively repeat forever. It is important to remember that not only are fractions like 1/2 and -2/3 rational numbers, but -5 and 100 are also rational numbers. By definition, a rational number can be written as a fraction, finite decimal, or repeating decimal. The number 5 can be written as 5/1 or 5.0.

The last subset of the real number system is the set of **irrational** numbers. By the process of elimination, try to think what this set must look like. We have discussed integers, fractions, repeating decimals, and finite decimals. Irrational numbers include the non-repeating decimals such as π and $\sqrt{2}$. It is important to note that there is NO number that is both rational and irrational. As the diagram on the previous page indicates, the set of irrational numbers does not intersect the set of rational numbers.

The set of **real** numbers includes both the set of rational and irrational numbers. (Note: The set of numbers that are not real are called imaginary numbers and involve the imaginary number i.)

Bringing it all together:

1. Name all subsets of the real number system which include 6/3.

   From smallest to largest: (recall that 6/3=2) counting, whole, integer, rational, real.

2. What is the smallest subset of the real number system that includes -7/8?

   It cannot be a counting number or whole number since it is negative. It is not an integer since it is a fraction that cannot be written as a whole number. So, the smallest set is the set of rational numbers.

Before moving on to operations, there is another concept that will be useful to mention. **Place value** refers to the position, or place, of a digit in a number. This position determines the value of the number. For whole numbers, place value starts at the "ones" spot and increases by powers of ten as you move from right to left as in the table below.

The place value for the underlined digit in each number is as indicated below:

Underlined Place	Name of Position
1,000,00<u>0</u>	Ones or units place
1,000,0<u>0</u>0	Tens
1,000,<u>0</u>00	Hundreds
1,00<u>0</u>,000	Thousands
1,0<u>0</u>0,000	Ten Thousands
1,<u>0</u>00,000	Hundred Thousands
<u>1</u>,000,000	Millions

Thus, thirty-four thousand, seven hundred ninety-two is written as 34,792. In expanded form, this number is written as (3 x 10,000) + (4 x 1,000) + (7 x 100) + (9 x 10) + (2 x 1).

Two hundred thirty-two thousand, one hundred four is written as 232,104.

Note there are zero tens, so a place holder of 0 is used in the tens place.

When performing the operations of addition, subtraction, multiplication, and division, it is important to pay attention to the place value. We will begin the discussion of operations by reviewing addition, subtraction, and multiplication for whole numbers.

To **add or subtract** 473,265 and 98,278, line up the place values as below.

$$
\begin{array}{r}
473,265 \\
+\ \underline{98,278} \\
571,543
\end{array}
\qquad
\begin{array}{r}
473,265 \\
-\ \underline{98,278} \\
374,987
\end{array}
$$

You might recall that when adding two digits, you must "carry the one" or regroup if the sum is greater than 9. In the case of adding 5 and 8 to get 13, the 1 (in the tens place) is regrouped so that it will be added to 6 and 7. In the case of subtraction, one can "borrow" from the preceding column, if necessary. In the above example, it is necessary to borrow 10 from 60 (a 6 in the tens place) before subtracting 8 from 5. So, one really subtracts 8 from 15 (10 + 5) to get 7.

To **multiply** the whole numbers 36 x 123, line up as below.

$$
\begin{array}{r}
123 \\
\times\ \underline{36} \\
738 \\
\underline{3690} \\
4,428
\end{array}
$$

Note that the second line in the calculation has a zero in the ones place. This is because the second step in the multiplication is to multiply the 3 in 123 by 30 (from $\underline{3}6$). As with addition, obtaining a product greater than 9 requires carrying the tens digit to the next column on the left. So, 3 x 6 =18. The one is then added to the product of 6 x 2. That is, 6 x 2 + 1=13, carry the one again. Finally, 6x1+1=7. Following these steps yields the complete first step in the above multiplication problem.

You can also multiply 123 x 36 by expanding 36 and using the distributive property.

$$123 \times (30 + 6) = (123 \times 30) + (123 \times 6) = 3,690 + 738 = 4,428$$

Many types of problems can be solved by performing operations with whole numbers. However, it will not always be obvious what steps should be taken. The table presented below shows some common key words that indicate addition, subtraction, multiplication, or division.

Key words to indicate addition, subtraction, multiplication, and division:

Addition	Subtraction	Multiplication	Division
Sum	Minus	Multiply	Divide
Add	Take away	Product	Quotient
Added to	From	Times	Divided by
Plus	Subtract		
Total	Remaining		

Three examples are given below. Try to determine the key words and use those to help you decide what to do.

Example 1: The ABC bus company needs to determine the number of passengers who ride their buses in a typical week in a certain city. The company decided to base their report on the number of bus riders they had during the first week of April. The number of bus riders for the days of that week were 2,132; 1,654; 2,017; 1,865; 1,702; 1,926; and 1,479. What was the total number of bus riders for the week?

Find the total number of bus riders by adding the numbers:

$$
\begin{array}{r}
2,132 \\
1,654 \\
2,017 \\
1,865 \\
1,702 \\
1,926 \\
+\ 1,479 \\
\hline
12,775
\end{array}
$$

Example 2: To find the **average** of a set of numbers, you must use the operations of addition and division. First, add the numbers in the set, then divide the sum by the number of numbers in the set.

In the preceding example, we found that the total number of bus riders for the first week in April was 12,775. To find the average number of bus riders per day, we divide the total number of riders by the number of days. Therefore, the average number of bus riders is 1,825 riders/day.

$$\frac{total\ number\ of\ riders}{number\ of\ days} = \frac{2{,}132 + 1{,}654 + 2{,}017 + 1{,}865 + 1{,}702 + 1{,}926 + 1{,}469}{7} = \frac{12{,}775}{7} = 1{,}825\ riders/day$$

Example 3: The ABC bus company finds that the average found in Example 2 is exactly the number of bus riders every day for 12 days in a row. The company has a goal of 25,000 bus riders for the two-week period. On the remaining two days, how many people must ride the bus?

This example requires two operations. First, you must multiply 1,825 and 12 (since multiplication is just repeated addition, 1,825 x 12 gives the same result as adding 1,825 twelve times). Next, subtract the product from 25,000 to find the number of riders for the last two days.

$$1825 \times 12 = 21{,}900$$
$$25{,}000 - 21{,}900 = 3{,}100$$

To meet the goal, 3,100 riders must ride the bus during the last two days.

Practice Problems

1. Subtract 98,765 from 257,143.
   a. 355,908
   b. 159,378
   c. 158,378
   d. 159,488

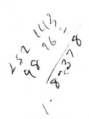

Use the chart below to answer question 2.

The annual budget for the Problem Solving Office includes the following expenses:

Employees Salaries	$184,000.00
Supplies and Postage	$ 9,745.00
Phone and Utilities	$ 6,300.00
Office Rent	$ 29,400.00
Travel	$ 12,570.00

2. Find the total of the expenses listed in the annual budget.
   a. $ 2,208,200.00
   b. $ 242,015.00
   c. $ 240,000.00
   d. $ 242,150.00

3. If $638,312.00 was the total income that a company expects for the year, and the total expenses listed in the annual budget were $248,165.00, how much profit would the company expect to make? (Profit is the total income minus costs.)
   a. $ 396,307.00
   b. $ 1,569,888.00
   c. $ 390,147.00
   d. $ 242,015.00

4. What is the average weight for four bears who have weights of 430 pounds, 374 pounds, 410 pounds and 390 pounds?
   a. 1,604 pounds
   b. 802 pounds
   c. 401 pounds
   d. 351 pounds

Solutions for Practice Problems (Whole Numbers)

1. c. The correct answer is 158,378. Line up the place values correctly. Remember to "borrow" as needed. You can check your work by adding 158,378 and 98,765.

$$257,143$$
$$-\underline{98,765}$$
$$158,378$$

2. b. The correct answer for problem 2 above is $242,015. Add all the budgeted items to get this sum. Remember to line up place values correctly.

3. c. The correct answer is $390,147. Subtract the total amount budgeted for expenses from the total expected income $638,312 – $248,165 = $390,147.

4. c. The correct answer is 401 pounds. Add the weights of the four bears and divide the sum by 4 to get the average weight of the bears.

Integers

Integers are the numbers {..., -3, -2, -1, 0, 1, 2, 3, ...}. The positive integers, also called the counting numbers, are the numbers {1, 2, 3,...}. The negative integers are the numbers {..., -3, -2, -1}. The number 0 is an integer that is neither positive nor negative.

The set of integers includes both the counting numbers (positive integers), their opposites (negative integers), and zero. Recall the diagram of the real number system. As you can see, all counting numbers are also whole numbers. All whole numbers are **not** counting numbers because the whole number 0 is **not** a counting number.

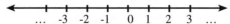

Observe that on the above number line, the numbers to the left of zero are negative. However, both a number *n* and its opposite, *-n,* are the same distance from zero. For example, look at the pair of numbers 2 and –2. Both are two units from zero (see diagram below). This distance from zero is called the **absolute value** of a number. Distance is always positive, so | -2 | = 2 and |2| = 2 where the symbol "| |" denotes the absolute value.

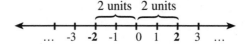

Adding and Subtracting Integers

A number line can help model how to add and subtract integers. Find the location of the first number in the addition or subtraction problem on the number line. For addition of a positive integer or subtraction of a negative integer, move right along the number line.

> *Examples:*
> 3 + 2 = 5. (Begin at 3 on the number line and move right 2 units.)
>
> 3 – (-2) = 5. (Begin at 3 on the number line and move right 2 units.)
> Note: 3 – (-2) = 3 + 2 = 5

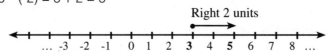

For addition of a negative integer or for subtraction of a positive integer, move left along the number line.

> *Examples:*
> -9 + (-11) = -20. (Begin at –9 on the number line and move left 11 units.)
> Note: -9 + (-11) = -9 – 11 = -20
>
> -9 – 11 = -20. (Begin at –9 on the number line and move left 11 units.)

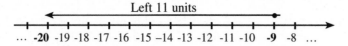

Another option is to consider the sign of each integer. There are two possibilities to ponder when adding integers; either the integers have the same sign or they have different signs.

If the signs of the integers are the same, add the absolute values of the integers and the result has the same sign.

> *Examples:*
> -9 + (-11) = -20 (Add 9 and 11. The result must be negative since both integers are negative.)
>
> 3 + 2 = 5 (Add 3 and 2. The result must be positive since both integers are positive.)

If the signs of the integers are not the same, subtract the absolute values and take the sign of the number with the larger absolute value.

Examples:

-9 + 11 = 2 (|-9| = 9 and |11| = 11. Subtract 9 from 11. Eleven has the larger absolute value and is positive. Thus, the result is positive.)

9 + (-11) = -2 (|-9| = 9 and |11| = 11. Subtract 9 from 11. Negative eleven has the larger absolute value and is negative. Thus, the result is negative.)

Tip: It is sometimes helpful to think in terms of money when adding integers. If you owe someone $13, but you only have $8, then you will still owe them $5 (-$13 + $8= -$5). Similarly, if you owe someone $9 and you have $11, then you will still have $2 after repaying the loan (-$9 + $11 = $2).

Subtraction of integers can be defined in terms of addition. In general terms, for any two integers x and y, $x - y = x + (-y)$.

Examples:

Original Problem	Rewritten as addition	Answer
3 – 7	3 + (-7)	-4
-5 – 2	-5 + (-2)	-7
4 – (−6)	4 + 6	10
-9 – (−8)	-9 + 8	-1

This table illustrates an important fact. Just as the opposite of a positive number is a negative number, the opposite of a negative number is a positive number. That is, $-(-n) = n$ for any number n. For example, $-(-7) = 7$.

Check yourself:

1.   What is the value of $-(-(-3))$?

2.   Add:
         -3 + 5

3.   Subtract:
         -9 - 13

Solutions:

1.   -3. Working inside out, $-(-(-3)) = -(3) = -3$.
2.   2. Subtract 3 from 5 and take the sign of the larger absolute value (in this case, 5).
3.   -22. This can be rewritten as -9 + (-13). Using the addition rules, add |-9| + |-13| = 9 + 13 = 22 and take the sign, -22.

Multiplying and Dividing Integers

To multiply two integers, multiply their absolute values. The sign of the product will be positive if the two integers have the same sign and will be negative if the two integers have different signs.

Problem	# of Negative Signs	Answer
-3 x 6	1	-18
(-2)(-4)	2	8
(-3)(-15)(2)	2	90
-1 x (-2) x (-5)	3	-10

Another way of determining if the answer is positive or negative might be clear from the table above. An even (e.g., 2, 4, 6) number of negative signs will yield a positive answer, while an odd (e.g., 1, 3, 5) number of negative signs will yield a negative answer.

To divide two integers, divide the absolute values of the integers. The rules for deciding if the answer is positive or negative are the same in division as in multiplication since division can be thought of as multiplication with fractions.

Problem	# of Negative Signs	Answer
12 ÷ (-4)	1	-3
-20 ÷ (-5)	2	4
-42 ÷ 7	1	-6

Order of Operations

When performing calculations with integers, you must perform operations in the correct order.

1. First, perform operations in **parentheses**. Work on the innermost set of parentheses first, then work outwards. [Example: $4 + (3 \times (\underline{5 + 2})) = 4 + (\underline{3 \times 7})) = 4 + 21 = 25$]

2. Second, simplify any **exponents**. An exponent is a way of denoting multiplication of a number times itself a designated number of times. For example, $6 \times 6 \times 6 \times 6$ can be rewritten as 6^4 and 8×8 can be rewritten as 8^2.

3. Third, complete multiplication and division from **left to right**. For example,
    $2 \times 8 \div 4 \times 2 = 16 \div 4 \times 2 = 4 \times 2 = 8$
    but, $(2 \times 8) \div (4 \times 2) = 16 \div 8 = 2$

4. Finally, do multiplication and division before addition and subtraction. Complete addition and subtraction from **left to right**.

Problem	Steps	Explanation
-2(3 - 5 + 2)	-2(-2 + 2) -2(0) 0	Subtract 5 from 3. Add -2 and 2. Multiply -2 and 0.
2 + 6 x 3	2 + 18 20	Multiply 6 and 3. Add 2 and 18.
(24 ÷ 3) x 5 - 6 + 2 x 7 - 3	8 x 5 - 6 + 2 x 7 - 3 40 - 6 + 14 - 3 45	Compute inside parentheses. Multiply and divide left to right. Add and subtract left to right.

Practice Problems

Perform the indicated operations in the problems below:

1. $(-3)(-2)(-5)$

2. $5 + (-1)(7 - 8 + 3)$

3. $(5 + 3) \times 2 - (4 - 5)$

4. $3^2 + 1$

5. $(3 - 1)^2 + 6 \div 2$

Solutions for Practice Problems (Integers)

1. -30. Recall that an odd number of negative signs indicates that the answer should be negative.

2. 3. Work inside the parentheses first. Inside, add and subtract left to right:
   $7 - 8 + 3 = -1 + 3 = 2$
   Then multiply by -1
   $(-1)(2) = -2$
   Finally, complete the addition:
   $5 + (-2) = 3$

3. 17. Work inside parentheses first. Then multiply, and then add.
   $(5 + 3) \times 2 - (4 - 5)$
   $8 \times 2 - (-1)$
   $16 + 1$
   17

4. 10. Recall that the exponent is a way of shortening repeated multiplication.
   3^2 means $3 \times 3 = 9$, so, $3^2 + 1 = 9 + 1 = 10$

5. 7. Work inside parentheses, then exponents, division and addition.
   $(3 - 1)^2 + 6 \div 2$
   $2^2 + 6 \div 2$
   $4 + 6 \div 2$
   $4 + 3$
   7

Rational Numbers

Recall from the diagram of the real numbers that the next set of numbers is the rational set, which includes the integers (whole numbers and counting numbers). As defined previously, a rational number is any number that can be expressed as a finite or repeating decimal. Below are some examples of rational numbers.

- $\frac{40}{5}$
- 7.999... (repeating decimal)
- -6
- -8.542 (finite decimal)
- $\frac{27}{4}$

Fractions

Fractions are numbers that can be written in the form $\frac{a}{b}$ where a and b are numbers and $b \neq 0$ (b is not equal to zero). The number above the line (a) is called the numerator, and the number below the line (b) is called the denominator.

If a number can be written in the form $\frac{a}{b}$, $b = 0$ with a and b integers, then the number is rational.

We generally use fractions when we want to indicate how many parts of a whole we have. If a cake is cut into 8 pieces and 2 pieces of the cake are served, $\frac{2}{8}$ is the fraction that represents how much of the whole cake was served.

If the numerator of a fraction is larger than the denominator, the fraction is an **improper fraction**. The **mixed number** form refers to the use of both integers and fractions to name the number. We simplify an **improper fraction** by changing it to a **mixed number**. This is done by dividing the denominator into the numerator and expressing the remainder as a fraction.

$\frac{8}{5}$ is an improper fraction. $\frac{8}{5} = \frac{5}{5} + \frac{3}{5} = 1 + \frac{3}{5} = 1\frac{3}{5}$

Two fractions are considered **equivalent fractions** if they are equal in value. To determine if two fractions are equivalent, simplify or reduce each fraction to its lowest terms (defined in the next paragraph). For example, $\frac{10}{20}$ and $\frac{4}{8}$ are equivalent fractions because both fractions can be reduced to $\frac{1}{2}$.

The **greatest common factor (GCF)** of integers a and b is the largest positive integer that will divide into both a and b. To **reduce a fraction to its lowest terms**, divide the numerator and denominator by the **greatest common factor** and determine if the final answer is positive or negative as shown in the examples below:

$\frac{12}{18} = \frac{6 \times 2}{6 \times 3} = \frac{2}{3}$ Six is the GCF of 12 and 18. Divide the numerator and denominator by 6.

$$\frac{24}{80} = \frac{8 \times 3}{8 \times 10} = \frac{3}{10}$$ Eight is the GCF of 24 and 80. Divide the numerator and denominator by 8.

$$\frac{-5}{-25} = \frac{5 \times -1}{5 \times -5} = \frac{-1}{-5} = \frac{1}{5}$$

Five is the GCF of -5 and -25. Divide the numerator and denominator by 5. A negative number divided by a negative number is positive. So the answer is $\frac{1}{5}$.

A **common denominator** for two or more fractions is an integer that is divisible by each of the denominators. To **add or subtract two fractions**, you must have a common denominator. If the two denominators are not the same, first find a **common denominator**. The fractions $\frac{1}{5}$ and $\frac{3}{5}$ have like denominators, and the two fractions $\frac{2}{3}$ and $\frac{5}{12}$ have unlike denominators. The denominators for the fractions $\frac{1}{5}$ and $\frac{3}{5}$ are alike, so we simply add the numerators to compute the sum: $\frac{1}{5} + \frac{3}{5} = \frac{1+3}{5} = \frac{4}{5}$

To add the two fractions $\frac{2}{3}$ and $\frac{5}{12}$, we must first find a **common denominator**. The smallest common denominator for the two fractions is 12: $\frac{2}{3} = \frac{2 \times 4}{3 \times 4} = \frac{8}{12}$

We change the fraction $\frac{2}{3}$ to $\frac{8}{12}$ and add the numerators 8 and 5 to get 13 as shown below:

$$\frac{2}{3} + \frac{5}{12} = \frac{8}{12} + \frac{5}{12} = \frac{13}{12} = \frac{12+1}{12} = \frac{12}{12} + \frac{1}{12} = 1\frac{1}{12}$$

Consider the problem $\frac{3}{8} + \frac{5}{6}$. The number 48 divides evenly into both 8 and 6, so 48 is a common denominator. Rewrite $\frac{3}{8}$ and $\frac{5}{6}$ into equivalent fractions with 48 as the denominator:

$$\frac{3}{8} = (3 \times 6)/(8 \times 6) = \frac{18}{48} \qquad\qquad \frac{5}{6} = (5 \times 8)/(6 \times 8) = \frac{40}{48}$$

Since the two fractions now have a common denominator, we can add them together.

$$\frac{18}{48} + \frac{40}{48} = (18 + 40)/48 = \frac{58}{48}$$

Since $\frac{58}{48}$ is not in simplest form, find the GCF of both the numerator and denominator. Divide both by the GCF, and change the answer to a mixed fraction as shown.

$$\frac{58}{48} = \frac{58}{48} \div \frac{2}{2} = \frac{29}{24} = 1\frac{5}{24}$$

Using the lowest common denominator (LCD), 24 we get:

$$\frac{3}{8} = \frac{3 \times 3}{8 \times 3} = \frac{9}{24} \qquad\qquad\qquad\qquad \frac{5}{6} = \frac{5 \times 4}{6 \times 4} = \frac{20}{24}$$

We determined what number multiplied times 8 equals 24. Since 8 would be multiplied by 3 to get the denominator of 24, we must also multiply the numerator by 3. Similarly, we multiply the numerator and denominator of the fraction $\frac{5}{6}$ by 4 to get the common denominator 24. To keep the value of the fraction the same, always multiply both the numerator and denominator of the fraction by the **same** non-zero integer.

Solving the same problem using the LCD: $\frac{3}{8}+\frac{5}{6}=\frac{9}{24}+\frac{20}{24}=\frac{29}{24}=\frac{24+5}{24}=\frac{24}{24}+\frac{5}{24}=1+\frac{5}{24}=1\frac{5}{24}$

Subtracting the fraction $\frac{3}{8}$ from $\frac{5}{6}$ works similar to addition. Find the LCD as above

$$\frac{5}{6}-\frac{3}{8}=\frac{5\times4}{6\times4}-\frac{3\times3}{8\times3}=\frac{20}{24}-\frac{9}{24}=\frac{11}{24}$$

It is sometimes necessary to subtract a fraction or a mixed number from a whole number. To subtract $4\frac{2}{3}$ from 7, change both to improper fractions. How do you decide what to use as a denominator for 7? Rewrite 7 so that the denominator is the same as the denominator of the fraction. Thus, rewrite 7 as something over 3 as shown:

$$\frac{7}{1}=\frac{?}{3}\text{ then }\frac{7\times3}{1\times3}=\frac{21}{3}$$

Next, rewrite $4\frac{2}{3}$ as an improper fraction. Remember that an improper fraction can be converted to a mixed number by dividing the numerator by the denominator and leaving the remainder in fractional form. So to go back to the improper fractional form, think about the process in reverse.

$$4\frac{2}{3}=\frac{4\times3}{3}+\frac{2}{3}=\frac{12+2}{3}=\frac{14}{3}$$

Now go back to the original problem. We want to subtract $4\frac{2}{3}$ from 7:

$$7-4\frac{2}{3}=\frac{21}{3}-\frac{14}{3}=\frac{21-14}{3}=\frac{7}{3}=2\frac{1}{3}.$$

Sometimes, it is more convenient to leave the answer in improper fractional form. In general, if the solution to a problem is an improper fraction or mixed number, refer back to the problem to determine the appropriate representation. If the problem consists of improper fractions, then the answer should be presented as an improper fraction. If the problem involves mixed numbers, then the solution should be a mixed number.

Check yourself

1. $\frac{4}{5}+\frac{2}{15}$

2. $3-5\frac{1}{3}$

3. $\frac{3}{15}-\frac{2}{25}$

4. $1\frac{3}{4}+3$

Solutions

1. $\dfrac{14}{15}$ The least common denominator for $\dfrac{4}{5}$ and $\dfrac{2}{15}$ is 15. So, multiply both the numerator and denominator of $\dfrac{4}{5}$ by 3 to get $\dfrac{12}{15}$. Then just add.

2. $-2\dfrac{1}{3}$ Change both to improper fractions with a denominator of 3.

    $3 = \dfrac{3}{1} = \dfrac{?}{3}$ Since the bottom was multiplied by 3, the numerator must be multiplied by 3. This yields a result of $\dfrac{9}{3}$ Similarly, $5\dfrac{1}{3} = \dfrac{5\text{x}3}{3} + \dfrac{1}{3} = \dfrac{16}{3}$. Finally, subtract: $\dfrac{9}{3} - \dfrac{16}{3} = \dfrac{9-16}{3} = -\dfrac{7}{3}$ or $-2\dfrac{1}{3}$

    Note: Since the original problem contained a mixed number, namely $-5\dfrac{1}{3}$, the answer should contain a mixed number (i.e., $-2\dfrac{1}{3}$, not $-\dfrac{7}{3}$).

3. $\dfrac{3}{25}$ There are two options for solving this problem. One is to find the least common denominator of 15 and 25 and continue as in Solution #1 above. This method yields a result as follows:

    $\dfrac{15}{75} - \dfrac{6}{75} = \dfrac{9}{75}$ This answer can be reduced since both 9 and 75 are divisible by 3: $\dfrac{9}{75} = \dfrac{3}{25}$

    The second method is to reduce $\dfrac{3}{15}$ to $\dfrac{1}{5}$ since both the numerator and denominator are divisible by 3. The problem is now $\dfrac{1}{5} - \dfrac{2}{25}$. The common denominator here would be 25 since both 5 and 25 divide 25. This method yields the same result:

    $\dfrac{5}{25} - \dfrac{2}{25} = \dfrac{3}{25}$

4. $4\dfrac{3}{4}$ As in problem 2, change both to improper fractions: $1\dfrac{3}{4} = \dfrac{7}{4}$ and $3 = \dfrac{12}{4}$. Both have a denominator of 4, so you just need to add the numerators:

    $\dfrac{7}{4} + \dfrac{12}{4} = \dfrac{19}{4}$. This should be changed to a mixed number: $4\dfrac{3}{4}$.

To **multiply two fractions**, simply multiply numerator times numerator and denominator times denominator. Then reduce the fraction to lowest terms.

$$\dfrac{5}{8} \text{x} \dfrac{2}{7} = \dfrac{10}{56} = \dfrac{2 \times 5}{2 \times 28} = \dfrac{5}{28}$$

We simplified the answer $\dfrac{10}{56}$ by dividing by the common factor 2 (2 divides both the numerator and denominator). Simplification can also occur prior to multiplication. For this example,

$$\dfrac{5}{8} \times \dfrac{2}{7} = \dfrac{5 \times 2}{8 \times 7} = \dfrac{5 \times 1}{4 \times 7} = \dfrac{5}{28}$$ since 2 is the common factor in the top and bottom.

Note: If one of the factors is a mixed number, first change the fraction to an improper fraction, then multiply.

To **divide two fractions**, rewrite the division problem as a multiplication problem by multiplying both the numerator and denominator by the reciprocal of the fraction. Essentially, this leaves a denominator of 1 and a multiplication problem to solve.

$$\frac{\frac{4}{5}}{\frac{2}{3}} = \frac{\frac{4}{5} \times \frac{3}{2}}{\frac{2}{3} \times \frac{3}{2}} = \frac{\frac{4}{5} \times \frac{3}{2}}{\frac{6}{6}} = \frac{\frac{12}{10}}{1} = \frac{12}{10} = \frac{6}{5} \qquad \text{Note that } \frac{4}{5} \div \frac{2}{3} = \frac{4}{5} \times \frac{3}{2}$$

As discussed, the division problem was changed to a multiplication problem by inverting the divisor, the denominator of the overall fraction. The shortcut for **dividing two fractions** is to invert the divisor fraction and change the division to multiplication. Thus for any two fractions:

$$\frac{a}{b} \div \frac{c}{d} = \frac{a}{b} \times \frac{d}{c} \qquad\qquad \frac{3}{5} \div \frac{6}{7} = \frac{3}{5} \times \frac{7}{6} = \frac{21}{30} = \frac{7}{10}$$

Check yourself

1. $2\frac{3}{8} \times \frac{2}{3}$

2. $\frac{5}{3} \div \frac{4}{15}$

3. $3 + \frac{2}{3} \times \frac{9}{10}$

4. $4\frac{2}{3} \div 6$

Solutions

1. Change $2\frac{3}{8}$ to the improper fraction, $\frac{19}{8}$. Now, multiply.

$$\frac{19 \times 2}{8 \times 3} = \frac{19 \times 1}{4 \times 3} = \frac{19}{12} = 1\frac{7}{12}$$

2. Use the reciprocal of the second fraction (always the one after the division sign) and multiply.

$$\frac{5}{3} \times \frac{15}{4} = \frac{5 \times 5}{1 \times 4} = \frac{25}{4} \text{ or } 6\frac{1}{4} \quad (\frac{25}{4} \text{ is the preferred answer since } \frac{5}{3} \text{ is improper.})$$

3. Remember the order of operations. Multiply and then add.

$$3 + \frac{2}{3} \times \frac{9}{10} = 3 + \frac{2 \times 9}{3 \times 10} = 3 + \frac{1 \times 3}{1 \times 5} = 3 + \frac{3}{5} = 3\frac{3}{5}$$

4. Change to an improper fraction, and take the reciprocal of the 6 to get $\frac{1}{6}$.

$$4\frac{2}{3} \div \frac{6}{1} = 4\frac{2}{3} \times \frac{1}{6} = \frac{14}{3} \times \frac{1}{6} = \frac{14 \times 1}{3 \times 6} = \frac{7 \times 1}{3 \times 3} = \frac{7}{9}$$

Ordering fractions by size can often be useful in solving real-world problems. To determine whether one fraction is greater than another, find a common denominator for the fractions. The fraction with the largest numerator is the greater fraction.

Example: Which is greater, $\frac{2}{3}$ or $\frac{3}{4}$?

$\frac{2}{3} = \frac{8}{12}$, $\frac{3}{4} = \frac{9}{12}$. *Hence* $\frac{9}{12} > \frac{8}{12}$, *so* $\frac{3}{4} > \frac{2}{3}$.

The following describes another method of determining which of two fractions is greater.

In the general case, let $\frac{a}{b}$ and $\frac{c}{d}$ be the fractions to compare, where a, b, c, d are integers and $b \neq 0$, $d \neq 0$. Multiply to create a common denominator, which allows for the comparison of the numerators:

$$\frac{a}{b} = \frac{ad}{bd} \text{ and } \frac{c}{d} = \frac{bc}{bd}$$

So, compare $\frac{ad}{bd}$ with $\frac{bc}{bd}$.

If $a \times d$ is greater than $b \times c$, then the fraction $\frac{a}{b}$ is greater than the fraction $\frac{c}{d}$.

Example: Which fraction is greater $\frac{4}{7}$ or $\frac{5}{9}$?

Since 4×9 is greater than 7×5,

the fraction $\frac{4}{7}$ is greater than the fraction $\frac{5}{9}$.

To compare fractions $\frac{a}{b}$ and $\frac{c}{d}$, simply multiply *ad* and *bc*.

Decimals

To **change a fraction to a decimal**, divide the numerator of the fraction by the denominator.

Example: $\frac{3}{8} = \frac{3.000}{8} = .375$

Divide 3 by 8 to get .375. Note: 3 can be written as 3.000.

The addition of the zeros does not change the value of the integer.

$$
\begin{array}{r}
.375 \\
8\overline{)3.000} \\
\underline{24} \\
60 \\
\underline{56} \\
40 \\
\underline{40} \\
0
\end{array}
$$

A **terminating decimal** is a number that ends, i.e., it does not go on forever. To change a **terminating decimal to a fraction**, consider the place values of each digit of the number. The place values for numbers written in decimal form reading from the decimal point to the right are shown in the example below.

.1	.01	.001	.0001	.00001
Tenths	Hundredths	Thousandths	Ten Thousandths	One-Hundred Thousandths

Thus, the decimal .5182 has 5 in the tenths place, 1 in the hundredths place, 8 in the thousandths place and 2 in the ten-thousandths place.

$$.5182 = 5 \times \frac{1}{10} + 1 \times \frac{1}{100} + 8 \times \frac{1}{1,000} + 2 \times \frac{1}{10,000}$$

To change the .5182 to a fraction, we write 10,000 as the denominator of the fraction (since 2 is in the ten-thousandths place) and the digits of the decimal as the numerator of the fraction.

$$.5182 = \frac{5,182}{10,000}, \text{which is then reduced to } \frac{2,591}{5,000}.$$

A **repeating decimal** is a number that repeats one or more numbers after the decimal point. These numbers never stop repeating. To **change a repeating decimal to fraction**, follow five steps:

1. Let n = the decimal number
2. Determine how many numbers repeat in the decimal. Raise 10 to the power of that number. (If four numbers repeat, for example, then raise 10 to the power of 4: $10^4 = 10,000$.)
3. Multiply both sides of the equation in step 1 by the number in step 2.
4. Subtract *n* from both sides of the equation.
5. Solve for *n*.

Example:

Step 1. $n = 0.33...$

Step 2. $10^1 = 10$

Step 3. $(10)(n) = (10)(0.33...)$
    $10n = 3.33...$

Step 4. $10n = 3.33...$
    $\underline{-n = -0.33...}$ (Note: n = 0.33...)
    $9n = 3$

Step 5. $n = \dfrac{3}{9} = \dfrac{1}{3}$

When **adding and subtracting decimals**, the place values must be lined up correctly. To find the sum of the numbers .2473, .025, .9, and 2.64, line up the numbers and decimal points as below and add.

$$
\begin{array}{r}
0.2473 \\
0.025 \\
0.9 \\
+\,2.64 \\
\hline
3.8123
\end{array}
$$

It may be helpful to add zeros to the right of the last digit in the decimal.

$$
\begin{array}{r}
0\ .2473 \\
0.0250 \\
0.9000 \\
+\ 2.6400 \\
\hline
3.8123
\end{array}
$$

The following is an example of how **decimals are subtracted.**

$$
\begin{array}{r}
3.106 \\
-\ 2.840 \\
\hline
.266
\end{array}
$$ (Note 2.84 can be written as 2.840)

When **multiplying decimals**, multiply as you would with whole numbers (ignoring the decimal point). Determine where to place the decimal point by counting the total number of digits to the right of the decimal point in the two numbers you are multiplying.

Multiply .34 x .216 as shown:
$$
\begin{array}{r}
.216 \\
\times\ .34 \\
\hline
864 \\
648\ \ \\
\hline
.07344
\end{array}
$$

Note: When you multiply, you get 7344, but we must count off 5 decimal places from the right to place the decimal. (There are two digits to the right of the decimal point in .34 and three digits to the right of the decimal point in .216 for a total of five. Therefore, we must leave 5 digits to the right of the decimal point.) A zero is placed in front of the 7 to get the fifth decimal place.

When **dividing decimals**, we generally change the divisor (or denominator) to a whole number as in the next example:

$$
\frac{.710}{.05} \times \frac{100}{100} = \frac{71.0}{5} = 14.2
$$

Note: The denominator had to be multiplied by 100 to change it to a whole number; we then had to multiply the numerator by 100 to keep the value of the fraction the same. The following is another division example:

$$
\frac{.8944}{.431} \times \frac{1000}{1000} = \frac{894.4}{431} = 2.07517 = 2.0752
$$

In general, round non-exact answers to the greatest number of digits to the right of the decimal in the original problem.

You can also use long division to divide decimals.

$$
\frac{.710}{.05} = .05\overline{).710} = 5\overline{)71.0}
$$

$$
\begin{array}{r}
14.2 \\
5\overline{)71.0} \\
5\ \ \ \ \ \\
\hline
21\ \ \\
20\ \ \\
\hline
10 \\
10 \\
\hline
0
\end{array}
$$

Rounding Decimals

To round a number to a decimal place value, look at the digit to the right of the place you wish to round to. When the digit is 5, 6, 7, 8, or 9, round up; when the digit is 0, 1, 2, 3, or 4, round down.

> *Examples: Round 1.726 to the nearest hundredth. We get 1.73 since the digit to the right of the hundredths place is 6.*
>
> *Round 43.621 to the nearest tenth. We get 43.6 since the digit to the right of the tenths place is 2.*
>
> *Round 22.629 to the nearest thousandths. We get 22.629 since the digit to the right of the thousandths place is 0.*

Practice Problems

1. George is making a gadget that requires $3\frac{1}{2}$ feet of red wire, $5\frac{1}{3}$ feet of green wire and $1\frac{3}{4}$ feet of yellow wire. How many total feet of wire does he need?
    a. 10 ft.
    b. $9\frac{5}{9}$ ft.
    c. $10\frac{7}{12}$ ft.
    d. 11 ft.

2. George is trying to estimate how much it will cost him to buy 3 ½ feet of red wire, 5 ⅓ feet of green wire and 1 ¾ feet of yellow wire. He calculates the total number of feet of wire and rounds the total to the nearest foot. If the wire costs $0.70 per foot, regardless of the color, how much is his estimated cost and how many total feet does he estimate?
    a. $ 7.20 for 10 feet of wire
    b. $ 7.70 for 11 feet of wire
    c. $ 72.00 for 11 feet of wire
    d. $ 77.00 for 10 feet of wire

3. Multiply 2.4 × .125
    a. 2.4 × .125 = .3000
    b. 2.4 × .125 = .0300
    c. 2.4 × .125 = 3.000
    d. 2.4 × .125 = 300.0

Solutions for Practice Problems

1. c. The correct answer is $10\frac{7}{12}$ ft.

    $$3\frac{1}{2}+5\frac{1}{3}+1\frac{3}{4}=3\frac{6}{12}+5\frac{4}{12}+1\frac{9}{12}=9\frac{19}{12}=9+\frac{12+7}{12}=9+\frac{12}{12}+\frac{7}{12}=10\frac{7}{12}$$

2. b. The correct answer is $7.70 for 11 feet of wire. When we round $10\frac{7}{12}$ to the nearest foot we get 11 feet. Multiply 11 x .70 to get $ 7.70.

3. a. 2.4 × .125 = .3000 (There is one digit to the right of the decimal point in 2.4 and three digits to the right of the decimal point in .125, so the final answer should have 1 + 3, or four, digits to the right of the decimal point.)

Algebra

In algebra, variables are used to represent numbers. Variables are represented by letters or symbols. To algebraically express the phrase "4 more than twice another number," we can represent the unknown number by x; then the phrase would be represented by 2x + 4. The number in front of the variable is a **coefficient**. The expression 2x + 4 is called an **algebraic expression**. (An **algebraic equation** has an equality sign. The equation 2x + 4 = 7 is called an algebraic equation.) Algebraic expressions contain variables or symbols often separated by addition, subtraction, multiplication, or division signs. Below are some examples of algebraic expressions.

$$x - 7$$
$$3 + 2x$$
$$\frac{x}{4}$$
$$37x$$

To evaluate an algebraic expression, substitute a numeric value for the variable and perform the indicated operations. Suppose we are given the algebraic expression $3x - 5$ and we are asked to find the value of the expression for $x = 4$. We substitute 4 for x in the expression to get $3(4) - 5 = 12 - 5 = 7$.

ADDING ALGEBRAIC EXPRESSIONS

Only expressions with the same variable(s) can be combined using addition and subtraction. That is, $2x + 5x = 7x$ (like terms) but $3x + 8y$ cannot be combined into one term because 3x and 8y contain two different variables.

Check yourself

Combine like terms to simplify the following expressions.

1. $2x - 5y + 7x$

2. $y - 3x + 4x + y$

Solutions

1. $2x + (-5y) + 7x = 9x + (-5y) = 9x - 5y$ Since the variable x appears with both a coefficient of 2 and a coefficient of 7, those two terms can be added together. That is, add two x's and seven x's to get nine x's.

2. $y + (-3x) + 4x + y = 2y + x$ Notice that the coefficient of x is a one. If the coefficient is a one, there is no need to write it.

MULTIPLYING ALGEBRAIC EXPRESSIONS

Multiplying algebraic expressions requires several steps. When multiplying a **monomial** (one term with no addition or subtraction) by a **binomial** (two terms separated by addition or subtraction), the monomial must be multiplied by each term of the binomial.

> *Example*: $3x(2x - 1) = 3x(2x + (-1)) = (3x)(2x) + (3x)(-1) = 6x^2 - 3x$

The property shown above is known as the distributive property. This property, in general terms, states $a(b + c) = a(b) + a(c)$

When multiplying a binomial by a binomial, the terms in the first binomial must each be multiplied by the terms in the second binomial. Tip: Multiply the terms that are placed first, multiply the outer two, multiply the inner two, and the last two—F(irst), O(uter), I(nner), L(ast).

> *Example*: $(2x - 3)(4x + 2) = (2x + (-3))(4x + 2) = \underset{\text{First}}{(2x)(4x)} + \underset{\text{Outer}}{(2x)(2)} + \underset{\text{Inner}}{(-3)(4x)} + \underset{\text{Last}}{(-3)(2)}$
>
> $= 8x^2 + 4x - 12x - 6$ *Combine like terms.*
> $= 8x^2 - 8x - 6$ *(Note: Always write the answer in terms of descending power.)*

$$(5x + 1)(x - 2) = (5x)(x) + (5x)(-2) + (1)(x) + (1)(-2)$$
$$= 5x^2 + (-10x) + x + (2)$$
$$= 5x^2 - 9x - 2$$

> *Note: Each term of the first expression is multiplied times each term of the second expression.*

When multiplying two algebraic expressions together, you may also solve the problem with the **area method**. To use this method, create a grid. Write the terms of the first factor across the first row and write the terms of the second factor down the first column (see the example below). Find the product (or area) of each inner box and then add all the boxes together.

	2x	-3
4x		
2		

Example: $(2x - 3)(4x + 2) =$

	2x	-3
4x	8x²	-12x
2	4x	-6

$= 8x^2 - 12x + 4x - 6$
$= 8x^2 - 8x - 6$

	5x	1
x		
-2		

Example: $(5x + 1)(x - 2) =$

	5x	1
x	5x²	1x
-2	-10x	-2

$= 5x^2 + 1x - 10x - 2$
$= 5x^2 - 9x - 2$

Equations involve two (algebraic) expressions set equal to one another. The following are examples of equations:

$$x + 7 = 13$$
$$2x - 6 = 10$$
$$2x - 7 = 3x$$

To find the solution to an equation, we use what are called inverse operations. The objective is to find the value of the variable. Inverse operations are used to isolate the variable on one side of the equation. To solve the equation $x + 7 = 13$, subtract 7 from both sides of the equation:

$$x + 7 = 13$$
$$x + 7 - 7 = 13 - 7 \quad \text{Subtract 7 from both sides}$$
$$x = 13 - 7 \quad \text{Simplify}$$
$$x = 6$$

The key to remember is that operations done to one side MUST be done to the other side as well. Note in the example above, seven is subtracted from both sides. Remember that subtraction is the opposite operation for addition, and division is the opposite operation for multiplication.

The following steps are used to solve the equation $2x - 6 = 10$:

$$2x - 6 = 10$$
$$2x - 6 + 6 = 10 + 6$$

Since 6 was subtracted from $2x$ we use the inverse operation of adding 6 to both sides. This eliminates -6 from the left side of the equation. To keep the equation balanced, we must do the same thing to both sides of the equation.

$$\frac{2x}{2} = \frac{16}{2}$$

Since x is multiplied by 2, we use the inverse operation of division to solve for x.

$$x = 8 \quad \text{The value of the variable is 8.}$$

Always check your solution by substituting the value you find back into the original equation. Since we found x = 8, we replace x by 8 in the original equation.

$$2(8) - 6 = 16 - 6 = 10$$

Example: Let x represent a number. The sum of x and ½ of x is 9. Solve for x.

$$x + \frac{1}{2}x = 9$$

$$1x + \frac{1}{2}x = 9$$

$$\frac{2}{2}x + \frac{1}{2}x = 9$$

$$\frac{2+1}{2}x = 9$$

$$\frac{3}{2}x = 9$$

$$\frac{\frac{3}{2}}{\frac{3}{2}}x = \frac{9}{\frac{3}{2}}$$

$$\left(\frac{\frac{3}{2}\times\frac{2}{3}}{\frac{3}{2}\times\frac{2}{3}}\right)x = \frac{9\times\frac{2}{3}}{\frac{3}{2}\times\frac{2}{3}}$$

$$\frac{2}{3}\times\frac{3}{2}x = \frac{9}{1}\times\frac{2}{3}$$

$$x = 6$$

Check by substituting 6 for x in the original equation.

$$6 + \frac{1}{2}(6) = 6 + 3 = 9$$

Example: *Carolyn bought 12 items for a total cost of $6.00. The 12 items consisted of cookies and candy bars. The cookies cost 60 cents each and the candy bars cost 45 cents each. How many cookies did she buy?*

Let x represent the number of cookies she bought. Since she bought 12 items, 12 - x would represent the number of candy bars that she bought. The cost of the cookies is .60x and the cost of the candy bars is .45 (12 – x), giving us the equation:

.60x + .45 (12 - x) = 6.00
(To eliminate the decimal, multiply both sides of the equation by 100.)

$$60x + 45 (12 - x) = 600$$
$$60x + 540 - 45x = 600$$
$$15x + 540 = 600$$
$$15x = 60$$
$$x = 4$$

Carolyn bought 4 cookies. She bought 12 - x = 12 - 4 = 8 candy bars.

Check: 4 + 8 = 12 items
        .60(4) + .45(8) = 2.40 + 3.60 = $6.00

Practice Problems

1. Jamal's age is 3 less that twice Henry's age. The sum of Jamal and Henry's ages is 39. How old is Jamal?
    a. 14 years old
    b. 39 years old
    c. 21 years old
    d. 25 years old

2. What is the solution of the equation $3x - 7 = 8$?
    a. $x = 2$
    b. $x = \dfrac{1}{3}$
    c. $x = 5$
    d. $x = 12$

3. If $y = 4x - 3$, what is the value of y when $x = -2$?
    a. 11
    b. -5
    c. -11
    d. 5

4. Combine the terms in the algebraic expression $3x - 2y + 7x - 5y$
    a. $\_xy$
    b. $10x - 7y$
    c. $3xy$
    d. $10x + 3y$

5. Multiply $(x - 7)(2x + 1)$
    a. $2x^2 - 7$
    b. $3x - 7$
    c. $2x^2 - 13x - 7$
    d. $2x^2 + 15x - 7$

Solutions for Practice Problems

1. d   Let $h = $ Henry's age, then $2h - 3 = $ Jamal's age.

    Add the two ages: $h + 2h - 3$ to get 39

    $h + 2h - 3 = 39$ Add 3 to both sides

    $3h = 42$

    $h = 14$ Henry's age

    Jamal's age is $2h - 3 = (2)(14) - 3 = 28 - 3 = 25$

2. c   Solve the equation $3x - 7 = 8$
    $$3x - 7 + 7 = 8 + 7$$
    $$3x = 15$$
    $$x = 5$$

    Check: $3(5) - 7 = 15 - 7 = 8$

3. c   Substitute − 2 for x in the equation $y = 4x - 3$

   $y = 4(-2) - 3 = (-8) - 3 = -11$

4. b   Combine the like terms $3x + (-2y) + 7x + (-5y) = 10x + (-7y) = 10x - 7y$

5. c $(x - 7)(2x + 1)$

   $x(2x) + (x)(1) + (-7)(2x) + (-7)(1)$

   $2x^2 + x + (-14x) + (-7)$

   $2x^2 - 13x - 7$

Percent

The word **percent** means per hundred. Thus, 20% = 20 per one hundred = $\dfrac{20}{100}$.

To **change a percent to a fraction**, remember that % means $\dfrac{1}{100}$.

Thus, $35\% = 35 \times \dfrac{1}{100} = \dfrac{35}{100}$ or $\dfrac{7}{20}$.

To **change a percent to a decimal**, divide the percent by 100. This can be accomplished by moving the decimal two places to the left and dropping the percent sign.

$$2.5\% = \frac{2.5}{100} = .025$$

Example: Change 23.5% to a decimal. $23.5\% = 23.5 \times \dfrac{1}{100} = \dfrac{23.5}{100} = .235$

To **find a percent of a number**, change the percent to a decimal and then multiply the decimal by the number. 32% of 150 = 0.32 x 150 = 48

$$
\begin{array}{r}
150 \\
\times\,.32 \\
\hline
300 \\
4500 \\
\hline
48.00
\end{array}
$$

Example 1   *A grocery store bought 300 red delicious apples. If 18% of the apples rotted before they were sold, how many apples were left to sell?*

Method 1   *First, find the number of apples that rotted by multiplying 0.18 x 300 = 54. Since 54 apples rotted, subtract that number from 300 to get the number of apples left to sell.*

300 - 54 = 246 apples left to sell.

Method 2   *An alternate method for finding the number of apples left to sell is to subtract the 18% that rotted from the total 100% to get 100% - 18% = 82% as the percent that is left to sell.*

82% of 300 = 0.82 x 300 = 246

To determine the percent one number is of another number, set up an equation as shown in the next example.

Example 2   *On Monday, 3 students out of a class of 24 were absent from class. What percent of the students were absent from class? Let a denote the number of students who were absent, then $\dfrac{a}{100} = a\%$. a % of 24 is 3, so we get $(\dfrac{a}{100})(24) = 3$.*

$$\frac{a}{100} \times 24 = 3 \ or \ \frac{24a}{100} = 3$$

$$100 \times \frac{24a}{100} = 100 \times 3$$

$$24a = 300$$

$$\frac{24a}{24} = \frac{300}{24}$$

$$a = \frac{300}{24}$$

$$a = 12.5$$

12.5% of the students were absent.

Practice Problems

1. 12 is 20% of what number?
    a. 2.40
    b. 240
    c. 60
    d. .60

2. The 18 students who received an "A" in a mathematics class made up 30% of the students in the class. Find the total number of students in the class.
    a. 18
    b. 60
    c. 30
    d. 54

Solutions to Practice Problems

1. c   12 is 20% of 60. Set up the equation 12 = .20x. Divide both sides by 0.20 to solve the equation and get x = 60.

2. b   Let x denote the number of students in the class. Then 30% of x =18, or .30x=18

$$30\% \ of \ x = 18$$
$$.30x = 18$$
$$x = \frac{18}{.30} = \frac{1800}{30} = 60$$

There were 60 students in the class.

Ratios and Proportions

A **ratio** is a comparison of two numbers by division.
A **proportion** is two equal ratios.

If the members of a club consist of 12 men and 17 women, the ratio of men to women in the club is 12 to 17 or 12:17 or $\dfrac{12}{17}$.

If a 3-gallon punch recipe serves 25 people, we can use a proportion to determine how many gallons of punch are needed to serve 60 people. We get $\dfrac{3 \text{ gallons}}{25 \text{ people}} = \dfrac{x \text{ gallons}}{60 \text{ people}}$

Now cross-multiply to get:

$$25x = 3 \times 60$$
$$25x = 180$$
$$x = \frac{180}{25}$$

$x = 7.2$ gallons of punch

As you will see while working through the practice problems below, proportions have many applications in everyday life. For example, proportions can be used to determine distance traveled and to change recipes to reflect a new number of servings.

Practice Problems:

1. Solve the proportion $\dfrac{3}{x} = \dfrac{4}{12}$.
   a. 9
   b. 1
   c. $\dfrac{1}{9}$
   d. 144

2. If you can travel 180 miles in 3 hours, how long will it take you to travel 300 miles at the same rate of speed?
   a. $1\dfrac{4}{5}$ hours
   b. 2 hours
   c. 5 hours
   d. 8 hours

3. The 4 members in the Fairview Community Club who do not know how to swim constitute 8 percent of the total club members. How many members are in the club?
   a. 32 members
   b. 50 members
   c. 46 members
   d. 12 members

4. If John can drive 130 miles in 2 hours, how far can he drive in 5 hours if he travels at the same rate of speed?
    a. 325 miles
    b. 650 miles
    c. 52 miles
    d. 390 miles

5. If 4 wait staff are required to serve 48 people at a banquet, how many wait staff are needed to serve 120 people?
    a. 2 wait staff
    b. 8 wait staff
    c. 10 wait staff
    d. 12 wait staff

Solutions for Practice Problems

1. a   The correct solution is 9. Cross-multiply to get $4x = 36$. Divide both sides by 4.

2. c   The correct answer is 5 hours.

    Solve using proportions:

    $$\frac{3\,\text{hours}}{180\,\text{miles}} = \frac{t\,\text{hours}}{300\,\text{miles}}$$
    $$180t = 900$$
    $$t = \frac{900}{180}$$
    $$t = 5$$

3. b   The correct answer is 50. Let m represent the number of members in the club.

    This problem can be solved by using a proportion.

    Set up the proportion $8\% = \dfrac{8\,\text{members}}{100\,\text{members}} = \dfrac{4\,\text{members}}{m\,\text{members}}$

    Cross-multiply to get 8m = 400, and solve to get m = 50. There are 50 members in the club.

4. a   The correct answer is 325 miles.

    Set up the proportion $\dfrac{2\,\text{hours}}{130\,\text{miles}} = \dfrac{5\,\text{hours}}{m\,\text{miles}}$ where m equals the miles traveled in 5 hours.

    Solve the proportion to get:

    $$2m = (5)(130)$$
    $$2m = 650$$
    $$m = 325\,\text{miles}$$

5. c   The correct answer is 10 wait staff.

To solve the problem, set up a proportion as shown with *w*, the number of wait staff needed.

$$\frac{4}{48} = \frac{w}{120}$$
$$48w = 480$$
$$w = 10$$

Inequalities

Inequalities are expressions that are not equal. The symbols for inequalities are:

< less than
> greater than
≤ less than or equal to
≥ greater than or equal to

The method of solving inequalities is similar to the method for solving equations. However, if you multiply or divide by a negative number, the sign of the inequality is reversed.

$$
\begin{aligned}
2x - 1 &\leq 15 \\
2x - 1 + 1 &\leq 15 + 1 \\
2x &\leq 16 \\
x &\leq 8
\end{aligned}
$$

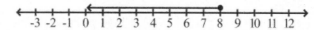

The graph of the solution set is shown above. The colored in circle at 8 means that 8 is a possible value for **x**.

Both the symbolic representation and the line graph indicate that the solution set contains all the numbers less than or equal to 8.

The solution set for $-3x + 5 \geq 17$ is found as follows:

$$
\begin{aligned}
-3x + 5 &\geq 17 \\
-3x + 5 - 5 &\geq 17 - 5 \\
-3x &\geq 12 \\
\frac{-3x}{-3} &\leq \frac{12}{-3} \\
x &\leq -4
\end{aligned}
$$

(The inequality reversed when we divided by a negative number)

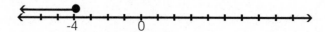

You can avoid dividing by a negative number if you add $3x$ to both sides as follows:

$-3x + 5 \geq 17$

$-3x + 5 + 3x \geq 17 + 3x$

$5 \geq 17 + 3x$

$-17 + 5 \geq 17 + 3x + (-17)$

$-12 \geq 3x$

$-4 \geq x$

The next example involves just greater than. This means that the values must be greater than the solution shown to make the inequality true.

$$2x - 3 > 11$$
$$2x - 3 + 3 > 11 + 3$$
$$2x > 14$$
$$x > 7$$

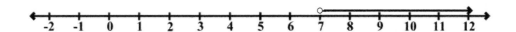

Note: There is an open circle at 7, since **x** must be greater than, and **not** equal to 7.

Practice Problems

1. Which of the answers below correctly describes the graph shown?

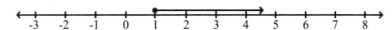

       a. x > 1
       b. x < 1
       c. x ≤ 1
       d. x ≥ 1

2. Solve -4x – 7 < 21.
       a. x < -7
       b. x > -7
       c. x < 7
       d. x > 7

Solutions for Practice Problems

1.   d.   The correct answer is $x \geq 1$.

2.   b.   Add 7 to both sides to get -4x < 28. Divide by -4. Remember to flip the inequality sign since -4 is negative! The result is x > -7. Alternatively, add -4x to both sides to get -7 -4 x + 4x < 21 + 4x. Simplify to -7 < 21 + 4.

        Subtract 21 from both sides to get -28 < 4x. Divide by 4. The result is -7 < x .

Formulas

Formulas are often used to solve algebra problems. Examples of formulas are:

Distance formula $D = rt$ *(distance = rate multiplied by the time traveled)*
Interest formula $I = prt$ *(interest = principal multiplied by the rate multiplied by the time, where r is a simple (not compound), interest rate)*
(Note: The "principal amount" is the amount initially invested.)

When solving equations involving formulas, substitute for values of the known variables and then solve for the unknown variable.

Example 1: *If $4,000 is invested at a simple interest rate of 4.5% for 2 years, find the amount of interest earned.*

We use the formula $I = prt$ to find the amount of interest earned.
$I = (\$4,000)(.045)(2) = \$360.00$

Example 2: *Suppose we know the amount of interest earned for one year was $150.00 and the simple interest rate was 6%. Find the amount of money invested.*

We know the amount of interest earned, the amount of time, and the interest rate. We must find the principal. $I = prt$

$$150 = (p)(.06)(1)$$
$$150 = .06p$$
$$\frac{150}{.06} = \frac{.06p}{.06}$$
$$\$2,500 = p$$

Practice Problems

1. If you travel at a rate of 55 miles per hour, how long will it take you to travel 330 miles?
    a.   5.5 hours
    b.   7 hours
    c.   5 hours
    d.   6 hours

2. How much interest will be earned on an investment of $5,000 invested for 3 years at a simple interest rate of 8%?
    a. $ 400.00
    b. $ 12,000.00
    c. $ 1,200.00
    d. $ 133.00

Solutions for Practice Problems

1.   d   Use the distance formula $D = rt$. Substitute 330 for the distance, D, and 55 for the rate, r.

$$D = rt$$
$$330 = 55t$$
$$t = 6 \text{ hours}$$

2.   c   Use the Interest formula $I = prt$. Substitute $5,000 for p, 8% = .08 for r, and 3 for t.

$$I = \$5,000 \times .08 \times 3 = \$ 1,200.00$$

Measurement

Measurements may involve English or Metric units. The basic units of measurements for both systems are provided here. Some equivalency measures for the two systems are also provided. The measures considered here are length, volume, and weight.

English units of Measurement

Length	Volume	Weight
inch	ounces (oz)	ounces
1 foot = 12 inches	1 cup = 8 oz	1 pound (lb) = 16 oz
1 yard = 3 feet	1 pint = 2 cups	1 ton = 2,000 lbs
1 mile = 5,280 feet	1 quart = 2 pints	
	1 gallon = 4 quarts = 128 oz	

Metric Units of Measurement

Metric units of measurement are based on multiples of 10.

Metric System Prefixes	
kilo	1,000
hecto	100
deka	10
basic unit (no prefix)	1
deci	.1
centi	.01
milli	.001

If the basic unit of measure is a liter, using the previous table you note that:

1 kiloliter	=	1,000 liters
1 hectoliter	=	100 liters
1 dekaliter	=	10 liters
liter		1
1 deciliter	=	.1 liter
1 centiliter	=	.01 liter
1 milliliter	=	.001 liter

The basic units of measurement for the metric system are meter for length, liter for volume, and gram for mass or weight. The prefixes for length, volume, and mass operate the same way. If we are looking at length, the table below would have meters as the basic unit.

kilometer	=	1,000 meters
hectometer	=	100 meters
dekameter	=	10 meters
meter	=	1
decimeter	=	.1 meter
centimeter	=	.01 meter
millimeter	=	.001 meter

Thus, 1 hectometer = 100 meters and 100 centimeters = 1 meter.

Equivalences of some English and Metric Units

The following are approximations of some English and Metric units:

1 liter	≈	1 quart (1.06 quarts)
1 kilogram	≈	2.2 pounds
2.54 cm	=	1 inch
1 oz	≈	28 grams
1 meter	≈	1 yard (1.09 yds)

Example: *How many inches are in 4 yards?*
There are 144 inches in 4 yards.
Since 1 yard = 3 feet = 3 x 12 inches = 36 inches.
4 yards = 4 x 36 inches = 144 inches

Example: *How many centiliters are in 10 liters?*
There are 1,000 centiliters in 10 liters.
l liter = 100 centiliters, thus 10 liters = 10 x 100 = 1,000 centiliters

Practice Problems

1. Complete the following:
    a.   3 pounds = ____ ounces
    b.   20 cups = ____ quarts
    c.   200 centigrams = ____ grams
    d.   3 kilometers = ____ meters
    e.   1 quart = _____ ounces

2. Approximately how many inches are in 12.75 centimeters?
    a.   32.385 inches
    b.   5.02 inches
    c.   32.385 cm
    d.   5.02 cm

3. How many inches are in $2\frac{1}{2}$ yards?
    a.   90 inches
    b.   10 inches
    c.   7.5 inches
    d.   30 inches

Solutions for Practice Problems

1. a. 48 oz (1 lb = 16 oz; 3 lb = 48 oz)
    b. 5 qt (4 cups = 1 qt; 20 cups = 5 quarts)
    c. 2 grams (1 gram = 100 centigrams; 200 centigrams = 2 grams)
    d. 3,000 meters (1 kilometer = 1,000 meters; 3 kilometers = 3,000 meters)
    e. 32 oz (1 quart = 2 pints = 2 x 16 oz = 32 oz)

2. b   1 inch = 2.54 cm. Use ratios to convert as shown below.

$$\frac{1 \text{ inch}}{2.54 \text{ cm}} = \frac{x \text{ inches}}{12.75 \text{ cm}}$$

$$12.75 = 2.54x$$

$$x = 5.02 \text{ inches}$$

3. a   1 yd = 3 feet = 36 inches. As in number 2, a ratio can be used.

$$\frac{1 \text{ yd}}{36 \text{ in}} = \frac{2\frac{1}{2} \text{ yd}}{x \text{ in}}$$

$$x = 36 \times 2\frac{1}{2}$$

$$x = 36 \times \frac{5}{2}$$

$$x = 90 \text{ in}$$

Distance between two points on a line

Suppose A and B are two points on a line as shown below. We find the distance between A and B with the formula IA – BI, where the bars represent absolute value. Distance is never negative, so we always use the absolute value. Since IA – BI = I- (B – A)I = IB – AI, one can subtract the value of B from the value of A and take the absolute value or subtract the value of A from the value of B and later take the absolute value. In the diagram below, the distance from A to B is 7 units since I10-3I = 7 and I3-10I = I-7I = 7.

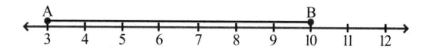

Practice Problem

If M and N have the values -2 and 12, respectively, find the length of $\overline{MN}$. (Note: $\overline{MN}$ means the line segment connecting M and N.)

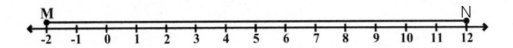

Solution for Practice Problem

The length of $\overline{MN}$ is $|-2-12|=|-14|=14$ units. Since distance always uses absolute values,

$|12-(-2)| = |14| = 14$ units is also a valid way of achieving the answer.

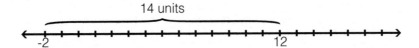

MIDPOINT BETWEEN TWO POINTS ON A LINE

The **midpoint** between two points on a line is the point exactly in the middle between the two points. It can be found by adding the two values and dividing by two. The midpoint between the two points, A and

B, can be found as follows: $\dfrac{A+B}{2}$. The midpoint has many useful applications in geometry and can be used in algebra problems as well.

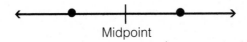

Practice Problem

Find the midpoint between -8 and 12.

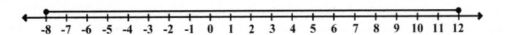

Solution for Practice Problem

Using the midpoint formula, $\dfrac{(-8+12)}{2} = \dfrac{4}{2} = 2$

Graphically,

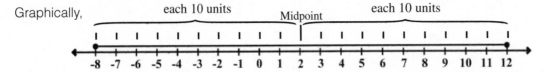

Formulas for Perimeters, Areas and Volumes

Circle

Circumference of a circle	$C = 2\pi r$	Where r is the radius of the circle
Area of a circle	$A = \pi r^2$	Where r is the radius of the circle

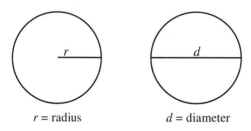

$\pi = pi \approx \dfrac{22}{7} \approx 3.14$ (3.14 will be used as an approximation for problems in this study guide.)π

The **radius** of a circle is the line segment connecting the center of the circle to any point on the circle. The **diameter** is the line segment that passes through the center of the circle and connects two points on the circle. The **circumference of a circle** is the total distance around the circle, i.e., the "perimeter" of the circle.

r = radius d = diameter

Triangle

Perimeter of a triangle	$P = a + b + c$	Where a, b, and c are the lengths of the the triangle
Area of a triangle	$A = \dfrac{1}{2}bh$	Where *b* is the base and *h* is the height

Note: The "b" in the perimeter formula represent the length of side b. The italicized *b* in the area formula represents the base of the triangle. Side b and base *b* are not always the same value.

Pythagorean Theorem

In a right triangle, the square of the hypotenuse is equal to the sum of the squares of the other two sides (called **legs** of the triangle). A right triangle has one right angle, an angle with a measure of 90°. The hypotenuse is the side opposite (across from) the right angle. In the formula $a^2 + b^2 = c^2$, the hypotenuse is denoted by the letter c and the legs of the right triangle are denoted by the letters a and b (see the diagram below).

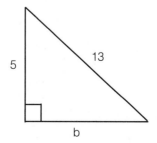

This formula is useful when given a right triangle where two side lengths are known. For instance, suppose one leg of a right triangle is 5 inches and the hypotenuse is 13 inches. The Pythagorean Theorem can be used to find the other side as shown:

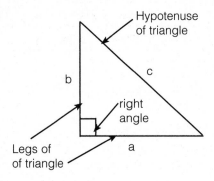

$c^2 = a^2 + b^2$
$13^2 = 5^2 + b^2$
$169 = 25 + b^2$ (subtract 25 from both sides)
$144 = b^2$ (find the square root of 144)
$12 = b$
$b = 12$ inches. So, the other leg of the right triangle is 12 inches long.

Rectangle

Perimeter of a rectangle	$P = 2L + 2W$	Where L is the length and W is the width of tl rectangle (Note: The opposite sides of a rectangle are equal.)
Area of a rectangle	$A = LW$	

Square

Perimeter of a square	$P = 4S$	Where S is the length of a side of the square (Note: All sides of a square are equal.)
Area of a square	$A = S^2$	

Volume

Cube	$V = LWH = S^3$	Length (L), width (W), and height (H) have the same measure, S.
Prism (box)	$V = LWH$	Length times width times height
Circular cylinder	$V = \pi r^2 H$	r is the radius of the base. H is the height of the cylinder.

Common abbreviations: sq. ft. = square feet; m = meter; " = inches

Practice Problems

1. Find the area of the figure to the right:
    a. 31.8 sq. ft.
    b. 60.0 sq. ft.
    c. 27.8 sq. ft.
    d. 48.0 sq. ft.

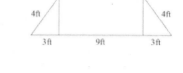

2. The shaded triangle is cut from a rectangular piece of fabric that is 10m long and 6m wide. What is the total area of the fabric remaining after the triangle is cut from the fabric?
    a. 30 sq. meters
    b. 60 sq. meters
    c. 16 sq. meters
    d. 32 sq. meters

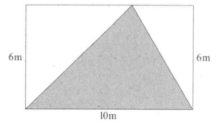

3. Last year, a farmer planted a rectangular garden that was 250 yards long and 120 yards wide. This year he plans to reduce the dimensions (length and width) of the garden by 40%. What will the dimensions of the garden be this year?
    a. 150 yards x 72 yards
    b. 100 yards x 48 yards
    c. 210 yards x 80 yards
    d. 350 yards x 168 yards

4. What is the perimeter of a rectangular garden that is 250 yards long and 120 yards wide?
    a. 30,000 square yards
    b. 740 yards
    c. 370 yards
    d. 15,000 square yards

5. How many cubic inches are in a box 5" wide, 3" deep and 8" long?
    a. 120 cubic inches
    b. 40 cubic inches
    c. 98 cubic inches
    d. 16 cubic inches

6. If the length of the line segment $\overline{AB}$ is 16 meters, $\overline{CD}$ is $\dfrac{1}{4}$ the length of $\overline{AB}$ and $\overline{AC} = \overline{DB}$. What is the length of $\overline{AD}$?
   a. 8 meters
   b. 12 meters
   c. 10 meters
   d. 6 meters

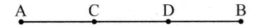

A C D B

7. Find the area of a triangle with a height of 9 inches and a base of 12 inches.
   a. 54 sq. inches
   b. 108 sq. inches
   c. 42 inches
   d. 21 inches

8. Approximately what is the circumference of a circle with a radius of 4 inches?
   a. 12.56 inches
   b. 25.12 inches
   c. 50.24 inches
   d. 4 inches

Solutions for Practice Problems

1.   a   The area of the figure is 31.8 square feet.
   The height of the triangle needs to be determined first. Use the Pythagorean Theorem to calculate the unknown side of the triangle (b).

$$c^2 = a^2 + b^2$$

$$4^2 = 3^2 + b^2$$

$$16 = 9 + b^2$$

$$7 = b^2$$

$$b \approx 2.65$$

Find the area of the two triangles and the area of the rectangle. Add the areas of the three figures to get the total area. The area of the two triangles are equal. Find the area by using the formula

$$A = \frac{1}{2}bh$$

Use the formula A = LW to find the area of the rectangle.

Area of the triangles $A = \dfrac{1}{2}(3)(2.65)$ *= 3.975 square feet.*

There are two triangles, each with an area of 3.975 square feet for a total of 7.95 square feet.
Area of the rectangle A = LW = 2.65 x 9 = 23.85 square feet.
Total area of the figure = 23.85 + 7.95 = 31.8 square feet.

2.   a   Subtract the area of the triangle from the area of the rectangle to determine the area of the remaining fabric.

Area of rectangle = (10m)(6m) = 60 square meters

Area of triangle $= (\frac{1}{2})(10)(6) = 30$ *square meters*

Area of remaining fabric is 60 – 30 = 30 square meters

3.   a   Find 40% of the length and width and subtract those amounts from the original length and width.
(.40)(250) = 100 yards (40% of length)
(.40)(120) = 48 yards   (40% of width)   *New length = 250 -100 = 150 yards*
New width = 120 - 48 = 72 yards
The new dimensions are 150 yards x 72 yards

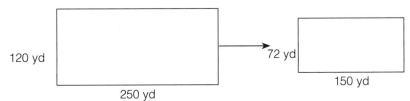

4.   b   Use the perimeter formula, P = 2L + 2W to find the perimeter of the 250 x 120 rectangular garden.
P = (2)(250) + (2)(120) = 500 + 240 = 740 yards

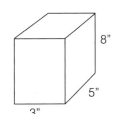

5.   a   Find the volume, V = LWH = (5")(3")(8") = 120 cubic inches

6.   c   If $\overline{CD} = \frac{1}{4}\overline{AB}$ *then* $\overline{CD} = (\frac{1}{4})(16) = 4$

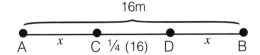

If $\overline{CD} = 4$ *, the remaining parts of* $\overline{AB}$ *must total 12, since 16 – 4 = 12*

Since $\overline{AC}$ *and* $\overline{DB}$ *have the same length, each must be equal to* $\frac{1}{2}$ *of 12*

Thus $\overline{AC}$ *and* $\overline{DB} = 6$ *. To get* $\overline{AD}$ *, we add* $\overline{AC}$ *and* $\overline{CD}$ *to get 6 + 4 = 10 meters*

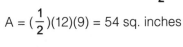

7.   a   The area of a triangle, $A = \frac{1}{2}bh$. Substitute h=9 and b=12 to get

$A = (\frac{1}{2})(12)(9) = 54$ sq. inches

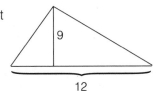

8.   b   The circumference of a circle is $C = 2\pi r$. So, substitute the approximation 3.14 for π and 4 for r to get:

$$C = (2)(3.14)(4)$$
$$C = 25.12 \text{ inches}$$

Graphs and Diagrams

There are many types of graphs used to solve problems. Graphs are visual summaries of data. Examples of some of the types of graphs and their interpretations are shown below.

Line Graphs show changes over a period of time. This graph shows the profits of Company A from 1995 through 2001.

- The company's profit in 1995 was $2,000,000.
- The company's profit increased from 1995-1997 and from 1998-1999.
- The company's profits decreased from 1997 – 1998 and from 2000- 2001.
- The company's profit remained constant from 1999 - 2000.

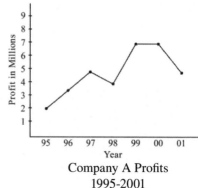

Company A Profits
1995-2001

Histograms and Bar Graphs are often used to show comparisons. The difference between the two is that the bars touch each other in a histogram and do not in a bar graph. In addition, the horizontal axes in bar graphs are normally labeled with words or categories. Histograms tend to be more quantitative.

This bar graph shows the number of inches of rain that fell in City X in the months of March, April, May and June.

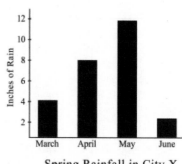

Spring Rainfall in City X

- 4 inches of rain fell in March.
- May had the greatest amount of rain.
- June had the least amount of rain.

Line graphs and histograms are created on coordinate axes. The **coordinate axes** are created by intersecting a horizontal and a vertical number line at 0. The horizontal axis is the ***x*-axis** and the vertical axis is the ***y*-axis**. To denote any given point, write the *x* coordinate and then the *y* coordinate as *(x,y)*. In the previous line graph entitled, "Company A Profits: 1995 – 2001," for example, the point (95,2) was created by locating the intersection of 95 on the *x*-axis and 2 on the *y*-axis.

Circle or Pie Graphs

To make a circle or pie graph, you need to know how much of the whole each part represents. Consider the example below of grade distribution in a health class.

**Grade Distribution for
24 students in a class**

A	4	$\frac{4}{24} = \frac{1}{6}$
B	6	$\frac{6}{24} = \frac{1}{4}$
C	8	$\frac{8}{24} = \frac{1}{3}$
D	4	$\frac{4}{24} = \frac{1}{6}$
F	2	$\frac{2}{24} = \frac{1}{12}$
Total	24	

The information at the left is needed to determine how much of the circle represents the number of students in each grade category. The angle measurement of a complete circle is 360.° The total of the angle measures for grades A, B, C, D and F must total 360.°

We will determine how many degrees each of the fractions in the table to the left represents. Note that there are a total number of twenty-four students in the class.

- The 4 students with As represent $\frac{1}{6}$ of the class of 24.

- The 8 students with Cs represent $\frac{1}{3}$ of the class of 24.

A	$\frac{1}{6} \times 360°$	=	60°
B	$\frac{1}{4} \times 360°$	=	90°
C	$\frac{1}{3} \times 360°$	=	120°
D	$\frac{1}{6} \times 360°$	=	60°
F	$\frac{1}{12} \times 360°$	=	30°
Total			360°

The circle graph below depicts the grade distribution for the students in the health class:

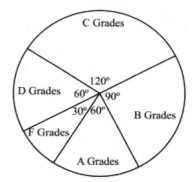

Grade Distribution
for Health Class

Stem and Leaf Graphs

Data is sometimes presented in the form of stem and leaf plots. The chart represents data displayed as a stem and leaf for the following set of data: 27, 21, 22, 21, 33, 31, 34, 45, 46, 41.

Stem	Leaf
2	7 1 2 1
3	3 1 4
4	5 6 1

The "leaves" are the unit or ones values and the "stems" are the tens values. Note that 21 appears twice in the data set and plot.

Practice Problem

The bar graph shows the average salaries of people in certain occupations. What is the difference between the lowest and highest salaries shown in the graph?

a. $ 40,000
b. $ 55,000
c. $ 25,000
d. $105,000

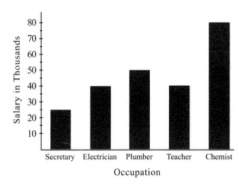

Average Salaries of
People in Certain Occupations

Solution for Practice Problem

b.   The chemist has the highest salary, $80,000.
     The secretary has the lowest salary, $25,000.
     The difference between the salaries is $80,000 - $25,000 = $55,000.

Statistics are commonly found in everyday reading. Newspapers often represent data in graphs and diagrams as well as in mean, median, mode, range and standard deviation.

The mean, median and mode are known as measures of **central tendency**. Often, people know that the **mean** is the arithmetic average of a set of data, and it can be found by adding the values of each data point and dividing by the total number of data points. The formula for finding the mean is

$$x = \frac{\text{sum of all data}}{\text{total number of pieces of data}}$$

$$x = \frac{x_1 + x_2 + x_3 + \ldots + x_{n-1} + x_n}{n} \text{ where n = total number of data points}$$

The **median** is sometimes used to find the central measure if the data contains **outliers** (data that are clearly different from the remaining data set). For example, in the set 17, 20, 16, 21, 22, 90, the outlier is 90. The median of a set of data is the middle-most value after ordering the numerical values from least to greatest. For an odd number of data points, the middle-most value is the median. For an even number of data points, the average of the two middle-most data points is the median.

The **mode** of a set of data is the number that occurs most in the data set. For example, 4, 5, 3, 4, 6, 7, 2, 4 has a mode of 4. If no number occurs more often than other numbers, the data set has no mode.

Practice Problems:

1. Find the mean, median, and mode of the following data: 5, 6, 1, 8.

2. Find the mean, median, and mode of the following data: 11, 15, 2, 2, 10.

Solutions for Practice Problems:

1. $\text{Mean} = \dfrac{5+6+1+8}{4} = \dfrac{20}{4} = 5$

Median = 5.5. (Remember, arrange numbers from least to greatest, 1, 5, 6, 8, and locate the number exactly in the middle. In this case, the number is in-between 5 and 6.)

No mode. All the numbers are different.

2. $\text{Mean} = \dfrac{11+15+2+2+10}{5} = \dfrac{40}{5} = 8$

Median = 10 (Again, arrange numbers from least to greatest, 2, 2, 10, 11, 15, and locate the number exactly in the middle.)

Mode = 2 (2 occurs the most often in the set of numbers)

Test Information

The Mathematics Practice Test you are about to take is multiple-choice with only one correct answer per item. Photocopy the answer sheet provided on this page to record your choices. Circle the correct answers on your answer sheet for each test item. When you have completed the entire test, you may check your answers with those listed in the answer key that follows the Mathematics Practice Test.

Mathematics Practice Test
Answer Sheet

1.	a	b	c	d	31.	a	b	c	d
2.	a	b	c	d	32.	a	b	c	d
3.	a	b	c	d	33.	a	b	c	d
4.	a	b	c	d	34.	a	b	c	d
5.	a	b	c	d	35.	a	b	c	d
6.	a	b	c	d	36.	a	b	c	d
7.	a	b	c	d	37.	a	b	c	d
8.	a	b	c	d	38.	a	b	c	d
9.	a	b	c	d	39.	a	b	c	d
10.	a	b	c	d	40.	a	b	c	d
11.	a	b	c	d	41.	a	b	c	d
12.	a	b	c	d	42.	a	b	c	d
13.	a	b	c	d	43.	a	b	c	d
14.	a	b	c	d	44.	a	b	c	d
15.	a	b	c	d	45.	a	b	c	d
16.	a	b	c	d	46.	a	b	c	d
17.	a	b	c	d	47.	a	b	c	d
18.	a	b	c	d	48.	a	b	c	d
19.	a	b	c	d	49.	a	b	c	d
20.	a	b	c	d	50.	a	b	c	d
21.	a	b	c	d	51.	a	b	c	d
22.	a	b	c	d	52.	a	b	c	d
23.	a	b	c	d	53.	a	b	c	d
24.	a	b	c	d	54.	a	b	c	d
25.	a	b	c	d	55.	a	b	c	d
26.	a	b	c	d	56.	a	b	c	d
27.	a	b	c	d	57.	a	b	c	d
28.	a	b	c	d	58.	a	b	c	d
29.	a	b	c	d	59.	a	b	c	d
30.	a	b	c	d	60.	a	b	c	d

Mathematics Practice Test

1. Multiply $2\frac{1}{3} \times \frac{5}{14}$

    a. $\dfrac{5}{21}$

    b. $\dfrac{5}{6}$

    c. $6\dfrac{8}{15}$

    d. $\dfrac{15}{98}$

Use information below to answer questions 2 and 3:

Brenda's take-home pay from her part-time job is $1,280.50 each month. She pays the following amounts for expenses each month:

Rent............	$350.00
Food............	$320.00
Utilities.........	$215.60
Transportation	$240.00

2. After paying the monthly expenses listed above, how much does Brenda have left for other expenses?
    a. $ 1,549.00
    b. $ 1,125.60
    c. $ 154.90
    d. $ 106.70

3. If Brenda spends the same amount for the listed expenses each month, what is the total of these expenses for a year?
    a. $ 1,280.00
    b. $ 1,858.80
    c. $ 13,507.20
    d. $ 15,366.00

This graph represents the results of a survey of 90 students regarding the types of exercise in which they regularly participate.

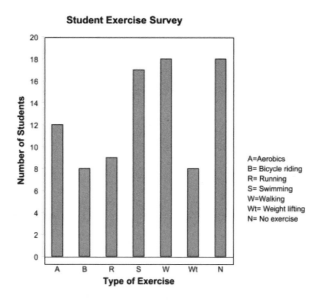

Student Exercise Survey

A=Aerobics
B= Bicycle riding
R= Running
S= Swimming
W=Walking
Wt= Weight lifting
N= No exercise

4. What percent of the surveyed students reported that they walk regularly?
    a.   .18%
    b.   18%
    c.   20%
    d.   .20%

5. Which answer is correct for the product .58 x .09?
    a.   .522
    b.   5.22
    c.   52.2
    d.   .0522

6. What is the median value for the set of data 20, 10, 16, 15, 12?
    a.   14.5
    b.   15
    c.   15.5
    d.   16

7. If 4 bottles of juice will serve 10 people, how many bottles of juice are needed to serve 35 people?
    a.   16 bottles
    b.   40 bottles
    c.   14 bottles
    d.   88 bottles

Use the information below to answer questions 8 and 9:

A menu at a deli lists the following items and their costs:

Hot Dogs........	$1.75
Hamburgers....	$2.25
Sodas............	$1.19
Potato Chips...	$ .99
Sandwiches....	$2.10
Cookies.........	$ .65

8. A customer bought 2 hot dogs, 1 hamburger, 2 sodas, 1 bag potato chips, and 3 cookies. How much did the customer's purchases cost?
   a. $ 11.07
   b. $ 8.93
   c. $ 13.17
   d. $ 6.83

9. Larry bought 3 sandwiches and 3 sodas. He paid for these items with a $20.00 bill. How much change was he owed?
   a. $ 9.87
   b. $ 10.13
   c. $ 10.23
   d. $ 16.71

10. Divide and simplify $3\dfrac{5}{9} \div 2\dfrac{2}{3}$.

   a. $1\dfrac{1}{3}$

   b. $\dfrac{24}{27}$

   c. $9\dfrac{13}{27}$

   d. $\dfrac{27}{256}$

Use the graph below to answer questions 11 through 13. The graph below shows the performance of Stock A and Stock B from 2000-2003.

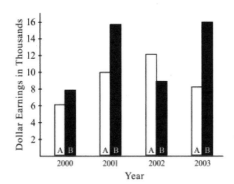

11. In what year were the earnings for stock B the smallest?
    a. 2000
    b. 2001
    c. 2002
    d. 2003

12. In what year did the earnings of stock A exceed the earnings of stock B?
    a. 2000
    b. 2001
    c. 2002
    d. 2003

13. How much more did Stock B earn than Stock A in the year 2003?
    a. $16,000
    b. $10,000
    c. $6,000
    d. $8,000

14. Given a segment $\overline{AB}$ with the length of 30 inches, what is the length of $\overline{CB}$ if $\overline{AC}$ is one-third the length of $\overline{AB}$?
    a. 10 inches
    b. 20 inches
    c. 60 inches
    d. 90 inches

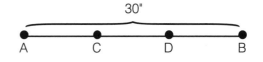

15. Express 5% as a fraction.
    a. $\frac{1}{2}$
    b. $\frac{1}{20}$
    c. $\frac{1}{5}$
    d. 1.05

16. A theater sold 480 tickets for a play last night. Floor seats sold for $30.00 each and balcony tickets sold for $24.00 each. The total amount collected for the 480 tickets was $13,200.00. How many seats of each type were sold?
    a. 200 floor seats and 280 balcony seats.
    b. 480 floor seats and no balcony seats.
    c. 280 floor seats and 200 balcony seats.
    d. 300 floor seats and 180 balcony seats.

17. How many centimeters are in 4 meters?
    a. 100 centimeters
    b. 400 centimeters
    c. 0.04 centimeters
    d. 0.4 centimeters

18. Find the total area of the figure shown.
    a. 60 square feet
    b. 54 square feet
    c. 72 square feet
    d. 30 square feet

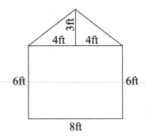

19. If it takes 4 hours to travel 240 miles, how long will it take to travel 90 miles?

    a. 1 hour and 30 minutes
    b. 40 minutes
    c. 10 hours and 40 minutes
    d. 22.5 minutes

20. Which algebraic expression best represents the following statement: Mr. Wilson's age, y, is 4 less than three times his daughter's age, x?
    a. x = 3y - 4
    b. y = 3x + 4
    c. y = 3x - 4
    d. x = 3y + 4

21. Order the four numbers shown from least to greatest.

$$\frac{8}{5}, \left|-\frac{12}{10}\right|, -\frac{4}{3}, \frac{4}{3}$$

a. $\left|-\frac{12}{10}\right|, -\frac{4}{3}, \frac{4}{3}, \frac{8}{5}$

b. $-\frac{4}{3}, \frac{4}{3}, \left|-\frac{12}{10}\right|, \frac{8}{5}$

c. $\frac{8}{5}, \left|-\frac{12}{10}\right|, -\frac{4}{3}, \frac{4}{3}$

d. $-\frac{4}{3}, \left|-\frac{12}{10}\right|, \frac{4}{3}, \frac{8}{5}$

22. If you purchase items that have a total cost of $42.20 before taxes, how much tax will you pay if the tax is 6.5%? (Round answer to the nearest cent.)
    a. $ 2.74
    b. $ 27.43
    c. $ 6.50
    d. $ 44.94

23. Gloria's scores on five tests in her mathematics class were 64, 80, 86, 72, and 88. What is the average of her test scores?
    a. 78
    b. 80
    c. 86
    d. 390

24. One circle has a diameter of 4 inches and a second circle has a diameter of 8 inches. How much larger is the area of the circle with the 8-inch diameter than the area of the circle with the 4-inch diameter (Use 3.14 as an approximation for π)?
    a. Two times as large
    b. Four times as large
    c. One-half as large
    d. One-fourth as large

25. Add and simplify $5\frac{3}{4} + 2\frac{1}{3}$.

a. $7\frac{4}{7}$

b. $8\frac{1}{12}$

c. $7\frac{1}{4}$

d. $8\frac{13}{24}$

26. Multiply the algebraic expressions $(x + 4y)(x + 2y)$.
   a. $x^2 + 8y$
   b. $x^2 + 6xy + 8y^2$
   c. $8xy$
   d. $2x + 6y$

27. How much interest would be earned on a money market account of $5,000 in two years if the annual simple interest rate is 7.4%.
   a. $ 740.00
   b. $ 370.00
   c. $ 3,700.00
   d. $ 74,000.00

28. The transactions Jermaine made in his checking account last month are shown in the table to the right. What was his checking account balance at the end of the month?
   a. $ 440.96
   b. $ 20.96
   c. $ 1,102.46
   d. $ 1,805.88

Debits	Credits	Beginning Balance
		$1,123.42
$ 247.16		
	$ 420.00	
$ 72.50		
$ 675.00		
$ 43.80		
$ 64.00		

29. Subtract and simplify $5\frac{7}{8} - 2\frac{9}{16}$.

a. $3\frac{1}{4}$

b. $\frac{31}{33}$

c. $3\frac{5}{16}$

d. $4\frac{1}{16}$

30. Multiply the algebraic expressions $(3x-5)(3x+5)$.

a. $9x^2 + 25$

b. $-12x + 25$

c. $9x^2 - 25$

d. $9x - 25$

Use the graph below to answer questions 31 and 32.

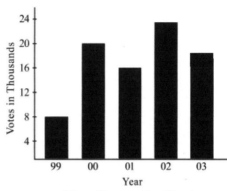

Voter Turnout in City A
1999-2003

31.   This graph shows the number of persons in City A who voted during the years 1999-2003. The city has 80,000 eligible voters. What percent of the eligible voters voted in 1999?
a.   10%
b.   25%
c.   50%
d.   .08%

32.   According to the graph above, the decrease in voters from 2002 to 2003 was:
a.   6,000
b.   16,000
c.   24,000
d.   8,000

33.   A certain cake recipe requires 3 eggs and $1\frac{1}{2}$ cups of sugar. How many cups of sugar are needed to make four times as much cake?

a. $5\frac{1}{2}$ cups of sugar

b.   6 cups of sugar

c.   4 cups of sugar

d. $\frac{3}{8}$ cup of sugar

34. Using the presentation of data to the right, write out the data set.

    a.   4, 7, 8, 9, 6, 3, 7, 7
    b.   47, 48, 49, 63, 67, 67
    c.   47, 48, 49, 63, 67
    d.   11, 12, 13, 9, 13, 13

Stem	Leaf
4	7, 8, 9
6	3, 7, 7

35. The temperature on a given day varied throughout the day from 8:00 a.m. to 5:00 p.m. as indicated in the graph. During what time of day did the temperature decrease?

    a.   From 8:00 a.m. - 11:00 a.m.
    b.   From 3:00 p.m. - 5:00 p.m.
    c.   From 11:00 a.m. - 2:00 p.m.
    d.   From 2:00 p.m. - 3:00 p.m.

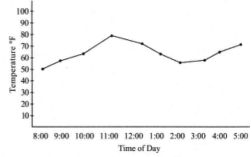

Daytime Temperature Patterns

36. Which of the following would you use to find the length, d, of the diagonal AB in the rectangle shown?

    a. $d = \frac{1}{2}LW$

    b. $d = 2L + 2W$

    c. $d^2 = L^2 + W^2$

    d. $d = LW$

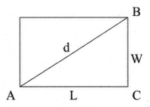

37. Perform the operations indicated to get the value of the expression. $6 \times (5 + 7) \div 4 - 7 \times 2 + 3 \times 3$
    a.   13
    b.   75
    c.   22.5
    d.   -72

38. Find the value of the expression 3x - 2y for x = 7 and y = 3.
    a.   5
    b.   27
    c.   -5
    d.   15

39. A technology fee of 3.5% of the charge is added to any credit card purchase. What is the total cost if the initial charge is $22?
    a. $7.70
    b. $0.77
    c. $29.70
    d. $22.77

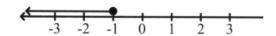

40. Which answer correctly describes the graph shown?
    a. $X < -1$
    b. $X \le -1$
    c. $X > -1$
    d. $X \ge -1$

41. What is the solution of the equation $\dfrac{x}{2} + 5 = 9$?
    a.   x = 8
    b.   x = 13
    c.   x = 5
    d.   x = 15

42. Evaluate the expression $2x^2 - 3x + 2$ for $x = 4$.
    a.   -2
    b.   6
    c.   22
    d.   54

43. Using the graph, determine the value of y when x = 4.
    a.   y = 4
    b.   y = -9
    c.   y = 6
    d.   y = 5

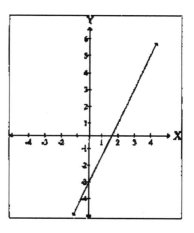

44. The grade distribution on an examination for a class of 30 students is as follows:

A	4 students
B	5 students
C	12 students
D	6 students
F	3 students

If a circle (pie) graph is used to represent the grade distribution for students in the class, how many degrees of the circle would be needed to represent the number of students who received a B on the exam?
    a.   30°
    b.   60°
    c.   5°
    d.   6°

45. Which algebraic expression below correctly represents the statement: One number, y, is 3 more than $\frac{1}{2}$ of another number, x?

    a. $y = \frac{1}{2}(x + 3)$

    b. $y = \frac{1}{2}x + 3$

    c. $x = \frac{1}{2}y + 3$

    d. $y + 3 = \frac{1}{2}x$

46. How many milligrams are there in 5 grams?
    a.   500 milligrams
    b. $\frac{1}{20}$ milligram
    c.   5,000 milligrams
    d.   50 milligrams

47. If 1 kilogram ≈ 2.2 pounds, how many pounds are there in 6 kilograms?
    a.   2.73 pounds
    b.   13.2 pounds
    c.   132 pounds
    d.   6 pounds

48. If the amount of interest earned in one year on an investment of $3,500 is $210, find the simple interest rate for the investment.
    a.   .06%
    b.   6%
    c.   .6%
    d.   60%

49. Divide the fractions and simplify your answer: $3\frac{3}{4} \div 1\frac{2}{3} = $ _____.

    a. $2\frac{1}{4}$

    b. $3\frac{1}{2}$

    c. $6\frac{1}{4}$

    d. $\frac{4}{25}$

50. What is the product of the numbers .23 x .045?
     a.   .1035
     b.   1.035
     c.   .01035
     d.   .001035

51. How much larger is $\dfrac{11}{12}$ than $\dfrac{5}{8}$?

     a. $\dfrac{7}{24}$

     b. $\dfrac{3}{2}$

     c. $\dfrac{4}{5}$

     d. $\dfrac{37}{24}$

52. A club has 9 male and 21 female members. What is the ratio of male to female members in the club?
     a.   3 to 7
     b.   3 to 10
     c.   4 to 10
     d.   7 to 3

53. The following amounts of beverages are needed to serve 72 people: 4 gallons of punch, 3 gallons of lemonade, and 2 gallons of tea. How many total gallons of these beverages are needed to serve 240 people?
     a.   9 gallons
     b.   30 gallons
     c.   240 gallons
     d.   80 gallons

54. Manuel has a credit card bill. A 1.5% service charge is added to the unpaid balance of the bill each month. If Manuel had a credit card bill of $1232.00, and he only paid $124.00 of it, how much would his new balance be after the service charge is added?
     a. $ 1126.48
     b. $ 1250.48
     c. $ 1108.00
     d. $ 1124.62

55. A circle with a diameter of 8" is cut from an 8" x 8" square piece of fabric. How many square inches of fabric are left after the circle is cut out (Use 3.14 as an approximation for π)?
     a.   38.88 square inches
     b.   50.24 square inches
     c.   64 square inches
     d.   13.76 square inches

56. Rain falling through a leaking roof filled a barrel at a rate of $\frac{1}{4}$ pints per minute. How many gallons of rain will be in the barrel after 12 hours?
   a. 180 gallons
   b. 22.5 gallons
   c. 48 gallons
   d. 1,440 gallons

Use the following diagram to answer questions 57 and 58.

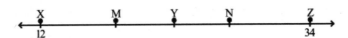

57. If point X on the number line is 12 and point Z on the number line is 34, what is the midpoint Y of the segment $\overline{XZ}$?
   a. 46
   b. 22
   c. 23
   d. 11

58. Given the segment $\overline{XZ}$ with a midpoint Y as shown above, where M is the midpoint of $\overline{XY}$ and N is the midpoint of $\overline{YZ}$, find the length of $\overline{MN}$.
   a. 5.5 units
   b. 11 units
   c. 28.5 units
   d. 17.5 units

59. A 4" wide by 6" long photo is enlarged 25%. What is the area of the new photo?
   a. 24 square inches
   b. 30 square inches
   c. 35 square inches
   d. 37.5 square inches

60. Kim drove 300 miles in 5 hours. How long would it take her to drive 125 miles at the same rate of speed (round to the nearest hour)?
   a. 12 hours
   b. 2 hours
   c. 1 hour
   d. 3 hours

END OF THE TEST

Mathematics Practice Test Answer Key

1. b $2\dfrac{1}{3} \times \dfrac{5}{14} = \dfrac{7}{3} \times \dfrac{5}{14} = \dfrac{35}{42} = \dfrac{5}{6}$

2. c   Brenda will have $154.90 left for other expenses.
   Add:

$ 350.00	
320.00	
215.60	$1280.50
+240.00	-1125.60
$1,125.60	$ 154.90

   Brenda's monthly expenses total $ 1,125.60. To determine how much Brenda has left after paying these expenses, subtract the total of the expenses from her take-home pay.

3. c   Add the listed expenses and multiply the total by 12 to get the total of these expenses for the year. 12 x $1,125.60 = $13,507.20

4. c   20% of the students reported that they walk regularly. 18 of the 90 students who were surveyed reported that they walk regularly.

   $$\dfrac{18}{90} = \dfrac{2}{10} = .20 = 20\%$$

5. d   The product of .58 and .09 is 0.0522. Remember to count the number of places to the right of the decimal.
   .58
   x.09
   .0522

6. b   Order the values from least to greatest: 10, 12, 15, 16, 20. Since there are an odd number of data points, choose the middle-most value.

7. c   14 bottles of juice are needed to serve 35 people. Use a proportion to solve the problem.

   $$\dfrac{4\,\text{bottles}}{10\,\text{people}} = \dfrac{b\,\text{bottles}}{35\,\text{people}}$$

   $$10b = 140$$

   $$b = 14\,\text{bottles}$$

8. a   The customer's purchases cost $11.07.

Item	Price	Quantity	Cost
Hot dogs	$1.75	2	$3.50
Hamburgers	$2.25	1	$2.25
Sodas	$1.19	2	$2.38
Potato chips	$0.99	1	$0.99
Sandwiches	$2.10	0	
Cookies	$0.65	3	$1.95
	Total		$11.07

9. b Larry would receive $10.13 change from a $20.00 bill.

Sandwiches	3 x $ 2.10	$ 6.30
Sodas	3 x $ 1.19	+ 3.57
		$ 9.87

To determine the amount of change, subtract the total spent from $20.00:

```
  20.00
 -9.87
  10.13
```

10. a The correct solution is $1\frac{1}{3}$. $3\frac{5}{9} \div 2\frac{2}{3} = \frac{32}{9} \div \frac{8}{3} = \frac{32}{9} \times \frac{3}{8} = \frac{4 \times 1}{3 \times 1} = \frac{4}{3} = \frac{3+1}{3} = \frac{3}{3} + \frac{1}{3} = 1\frac{1}{3}$

11. a The earnings for Stock B were the smallest in the year 2000.

12. c The earnings of Stock A exceeded the earnings of Stock B in the year 2002.

13. d Stock B earned $8,000 more than Stock A in the year 2000.
       Stock A earned $8,000 and Stock B earned $16,000. (Note that the graph indicates that the earnings are in thousands.)
       $16,000 - $8,000 = $8,000

14. b The length of $\overline{CB}$ is 20 inches. If $\overline{AC}$ is one-third the length of $\overline{AB}$,

$$\overline{AC} = \frac{1}{3} \times 30 = 10 \; inches$$
$$\overline{CB} = \overline{AB} - \overline{AC} = 30 - 10 = 20 \; inches$$

15. b $5\% = 5 \times \frac{1}{100} = \frac{5}{100} = \frac{1}{20}$

16. c There were 280 floor seats and 200 balcony seats sold.
       Let f = Number of floor tickets sold.
       Then 480 - f = Number of balcony tickets sold.
       30f = Total cost of the floor tickets.
       24 (480 - f) = Total cost of the balcony tickets.
       30f + 24 (480 - f) = $13,200.00
       30f + 11,520 – 24f = 13,200
       6f = 13,200 – 11,520
       6f = 1680
       f = 280 floor seats
       480 - f = 480 - 280 = 200 balcony seats

17. b 4 meters = 400 centimeters; 1 meter = 100 centimeters
       4 meters = 4 x 100 = 400 centimeters

18. a   The total area of the figure is 60 square feet.
To find the total area of the figure, find the area of the rectangle and the area of the two triangles.
Area of rectangle = 6 x 8 = 48 square feet
Area of the triangle = ½(4 × 3) = 6 square feet
There are two triangles with an area of 6 square feet.
The total area = 48 + 6 + 6 = 60 square feet.

19. a   It will take 1 hour and 30 minutes to travel 90 miles.

$$\frac{4 \text{ hours}}{240 \text{ miles}} = \frac{h \text{ hours}}{90 \text{ miles}}$$

$$240h = 360$$

$$\frac{240h}{240} = \frac{360}{240}$$

$$h = \frac{360}{240} = \frac{3}{2} = 1\frac{1}{2} \text{ hours}$$

20. c   The correct answer is $y = 3x - 4$.

$x =$ daughter's age, $y = 3x - 4$ = Mr. Wilson's age

21. d   Change each fraction to have a common denominator. In this case, it would be 15.

$-\dfrac{4}{3} = -\dfrac{20}{15}$ is less than $-\dfrac{12}{10} = \dfrac{6}{5} = \dfrac{18}{15}$

is less than $\dfrac{4}{3} = \dfrac{20}{15}$ is less than

$\dfrac{8}{5} = \dfrac{24}{15}$.

22. a   The tax amount is $2.74.

```
  $  42.20
  x   .065   (Change 6.5% to a decimal)
     21100
     25320
  $2.74300   (Rounded to the nearest cent)
```

23. a 78 is the average of Gloria's test scores.

$$\frac{64+80+86+72+88}{5}=\frac{390}{5}=78$$

24. b Four times as large

The area of the circle with a 4" diameter is $A=\pi r^2=3.14\times 2^2=3.14\times 4=12.56$

The area of the circle with a 8" diameter is $A=\pi r^2=3.14\times 4^2=3.14\times 16=50.24$

$\dfrac{50.24}{12.56}=4$, so the area of the circle with the 8" diameter is four times as large as the circle with

the diameter of 4". (Recall that the radius $r=\dfrac{1}{2}$ the diameter)

25. b $5\dfrac{3}{4}+2\dfrac{1}{3}=\dfrac{23}{4}+\dfrac{7}{3}=\dfrac{69}{12}+\dfrac{28}{12}=\dfrac{97}{12}$ or $8\dfrac{1}{12}$

26. b $(x+4y)(x+2y)=$

	x	$4y$
x	x^2	$4xy$
$2y$	$2xy$	$3y^2$

$= x^2+2xy+4xy+8y^2 = x^2+6xy+8y^2$

27. a $740.00 would be the amount of interest earned.

$I=PRT=\$5000\times.074\times 2=\$740.00$

28. a $440.96 is his balance at the end of the month.
Add the deposit (credit) to the beginning balance:
$1,123.42 + $420.00 = $1,543.42

Add the debits and subtract from the credits:
$247.16 + $72.50 + $675.00 + $43.80 + $64.00 = $1,102.46
$1,543.42 - $1,102.46 = $440.96

29. c $5\dfrac{7}{8}-2\dfrac{9}{16}=\dfrac{47}{8}-\dfrac{41}{16}=\dfrac{94}{16}-\dfrac{41}{16}=\dfrac{53}{16}$ or $3\dfrac{5}{16}$

30. c $(3x-5)(3x+5)$

	$3x$	-5
$3x$	$9x^2$	$-15x$
5	$15x$	-25

$= 9x^2+15x-15x-25 = 9x^2-25$

31. a The correct answer is 10%.
8,000 voters voted in 1999.

Thus $\dfrac{8,000}{80,000}=\dfrac{1}{10}=10\%$ of the eligible voters voted.

32. a   The number of voters decreased by 6,000 between the years
2002 and 2003. There were 24,000 voters in 2002 and 18,000
voters in 2003.
24,000 - 18,000 = 6,000

33. b   6 cups of sugar are required

$$1\frac{1}{2} = \frac{3}{2}$$

$$\frac{\dfrac{3\ \text{cups of sugar}}{2}}{1} = \frac{x\ \text{cups of sugar}}{4\ \text{cakes}}$$

$$(4)(\frac{3}{2}) = x = 6\ \text{cups of sugar}$$

34. b   Recall the definition of a stem and leaf graph.

35. c   The temperature decreased from 11:00 a.m. to 2:00 p.m.

36. c   The correct answer is $L^2 + W^2 = d^2$.
Triangle ABC is a right triangle with the hypotenuse, d. Then the Pythagorean
theorem holds $d^2 = L^2 + W^2$

37. a $6 \times (5+7) \div 4 - 7 \times 2 + 3 \times 3$

$6 \times 12 \div 4 - 7 \times 2 + 3 \times 3$

$18 - 14 + 9$

13

38. d   3x - 2y = 15 Substitute the values of x and y in the expression:
$3x - 2y = 3(7) - 2(3) = 21 - 6 = 15$

39. d   Change 3.5% to a decimal, 0.035. Multiply 22 x 0.035 = 0.77. Then, just add 22.00 and
0.77 (line up the decimals) to get $22.77. Another method is to multiply 22 x 1.035 = 22.77.
This works because you are adding tax to the original charge.

40. b   The correct answer is $x \le -1$.

41. a $\frac{x}{2} + 5 = 9$, $x + 10 = 18$, $x = 8$ (multiply the equation by 2), OR

$\frac{x}{2} + 5 - 5 = 9 - 5$

$\frac{x}{2} = 4$ so that $x = 8$

42. c   Substitute 4 for x in the expression $2x^2 - 3x + 2$

$2(4^2) - 3(4) + 2 = 2 \times 16 - 12 + 2 = 32 - 12 + 2 = 22$

95

43.　d　The correct answer is 5.　y = 5 when x = 4.

44.　b　The correct answer is 60°.　5 of the 30 students made grades of B.

$\dfrac{5}{30} = \dfrac{1}{6}$ Thus $\dfrac{1}{6}$ of the circle is needed to represent the number of students who made B's.

Since a circle has 360°, we find $\dfrac{1}{6} \times 360° = 60°$.

45.　b　The correct answer is $y = \dfrac{1}{2}x + 3$.

46.　c　1,000 milligrams = 1 gram

5 grams = 5 x 1,000 = 5,000 milligrams

$\dfrac{1}{1,000} = \dfrac{5}{x}$ so that $x = 5,000$

47.　b　There are 13.2 pounds in 6 kilograms
1 kilogram = 2.2 lbs

$$\dfrac{1}{2.2} = \dfrac{6}{x}$$
$$x = 6(2.2)$$
$$x = 13.2$$

48.　b　The interest rate is 6%.

$I = PRT$
$\$210 = \$3500 \times R \times 1$
$\$210 = 3500R$
$\dfrac{210}{3500} = R = \dfrac{3}{50} = .06 = 6\%$

49.　a　The correct answer is $2\dfrac{1}{4}$.

$$3\dfrac{1}{4} \div 1\dfrac{2}{3} = \dfrac{15}{4} \div \dfrac{5}{3} = \dfrac{15}{4} \times \dfrac{3}{5} = \dfrac{9}{4} = 2\dfrac{1}{4}$$

50.　c　23 x .045 = .01035
.045
x.23
135
90
.01035

51. a $\dfrac{11}{12}$ is $\dfrac{7}{24}$ larger than $\dfrac{5}{8}$

$$\dfrac{11}{12} - \dfrac{5}{8} = \dfrac{22}{24} - \dfrac{15}{24} = \dfrac{7}{24}$$

52. a   The ratio of male to female club members is $\dfrac{9}{21} = \dfrac{3}{7}$ The ratio is 3 to 7.

53. b   30 total gallons are required to serve 240 people.
         4 + 3 + 2 = 9 gallons required to serve 72 people.

$$\dfrac{9}{72} = \dfrac{x}{240}$$
$$72x = 9(240)$$
$$72x = 2160$$
$$x = 30 \text{ gallons}$$

54. d   The new balance will be $1,124.62.
         Subtract the $124.00 payment from the balance and add the service charge:
         $1,232 - $124 = $1,108 balance before service charge
         $1,108 x .015 = $16.62 amount of service charge
         $1,108 + $16.62 = $1,124.62 new balance

55. d   There would be 13.76 sq. inches left.
         Area of the square
         $A = 8^2 = 64$ sq inches

         Area of the circle
         $A = \pi r^2 = 3.14 \times 4^2 = 3.14 \times 16 = 50.24$ sq inches
         $64 - 50.24 = 13.76$ sq inches

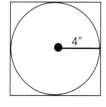

56. b   There would be 22.5 gallons in the barrel after 12 hours.
         1 gallon = 4 quarts = 4 x 2 = 8 pints

$$\dfrac{1}{4}\text{ pint/min} = \dfrac{1}{4} \times 60 = 15 \text{ pints per hour}$$
$$15 \times 12 = 180 \text{ pints in 12 hours}$$
$$180 \text{ pints} = \dfrac{180}{8} \text{ gallons} = 22.5 \text{ gallons}$$

57. c   The midpoint is 23. Using the midpoint formula, $\dfrac{12 + 34}{2} = \dfrac{46}{2} = 23$

58. b $\overline{MN}$ = 11 units

The midpoint of $\overline{XZ}$ is 23
The midpoint of $\overline{XY}$ is 17.5
The midpoint of $\overline{YZ}$ is 28.5
$\overline{MN}$ = 28.5 - 17.5 = 11 units

59. d   Since the width and length are both increased by 25%, multiply both 4 and 6 by 1.25.

$6 \times 1.25 = 7.5$

$4 \times 1.25 = 5$

Then, multiply the length times the width.

$7.5 \times 5 = 37.5$ square inches

60. b $\dfrac{300}{5} = \dfrac{125}{x}$

$300x = 625$

$x = 2.08$

The answer needs to be rounded to the nearest hour.
So, it will take her approximately 2 hours.

Section IV: Science and Technical Reasoning

The Science portion of the TEAS™ includes science reasoning, life science, human body science, chemical science, physical science, and general science. In this study manual, the subject categories have been separated for purposes of identifying major concepts, however, it is necessary to discuss various aspects of the subjects simultaneously. So, you may find that some topics are mentioned in association with other subject categories.

The groupings for each subject were mentioned earlier in this study manual. Recall that life science includes living systems, replication, and evolution among other topics. In human body science, the discussion will include information on the seven systems of the human body. Physical and chemical sciences are foundational to biological science. Chemical science will focus on such themes as atomic structure, compounds, and solutions. Physical science includes information on force and motion among other topics.

The ability to reason in science is a very important skill. It is something that cannot be taught on its own. Therefore, science reasoning is integrated into each subject area. Science reasoning allows you to apply scientific methods to given situations and to discuss scientific problems not immediately related to your surroundings. As you move through this section of the review, develop your ability to reason scientifically by going beyond memorization of the information. Question what is presented, try to develop scenarios on which to apply the facts, and look outside this manual for ways to use what you have learned.

Scientific Method

The goal of science research is to solve a problem or answer a question. Scientists attempt to achieve either goal by following a few basic steps.

1. Observe and determine the problem.
2. Ask questions and attempt to formulate a solution to a problem.
3. Collect data throughout the scientific process. Repeatedly, scientists gather as much information as possible in an attempt to answer the original question posed as well as new questions that occur as data are collected. Data are gathered utilizing four steps.
   a. Observation is a very important part of the process. Scientists utilize the five senses to learn as much as possible in the data gathering process. Observation can be direct, such as listening to a bird call, or indirect, such as observing qualities of other planets.
   b. Measurement is another part of data collection. Measuring allows for collection of quantitative (numerical) data.
   c. Data typically cannot be gathered from every member of a population. So, scientists collect information from a representative sample of the population. This means that scientists get data from a subset of the population that looks like the population, but is smaller and more manageable.
   d. It is very important for data to be organized in some way. This could involve putting information in tables and charts.
4. Formulate explanations to answer the questions asked in step 2. These explanations are called hypotheses. Hypotheses involve making predictions that follow from the initial statement of the problem. These predictions are then tested through experimentation.
5. Test the hypotheses or predictions in a controlled environment. Experimentation involves comparing a control group and an experimental group. The two groups both represent the population equally well. The difference is that the experimental group is given some type of treatment, or is different from the control group on one variable. Both groups are compared to see what effect the treatment is having on the experimental group. That is, the experiment tests the question, "What effect is the

independent variable (treatment) having on the dependent variable (the actions in both groups being compared)?"

    a. Scientists must then analyze the data gathered during experimentation. The researchers must determine if the data are reliable (consistent with past results) and whether the data support the hypotheses.

    b. Comparisons of patient groups in clinical studies are complicated by additional differences between the groups in gender, age, lifestyle, and other hard-to-control factors. However, the basic experimental protocol remains at the core of modern medical research.

6. The purpose of the scientific process is to develop a conclusion. Scientists produce models to represent the explanation supported by the data.

    a. Inference is used quite often in scientific research. Inference is a way of drawing conclusions without direct observation.

    b. After many experiments and model development, it is possible to develop a theory about a particular event. This is a broad statement of what is thought to be true. Note that it is always possible to find information that may refute a theory. So, a theory is thought to be true, but it might be proven incorrect when technology enables better data collection.

Life Science

The main purposes of life science are to understand and explain the nature of life. Life science includes the study of cells, organisms, ecology, and evolution. Biology is the study of all living things from very small structures such as cells to interactions of groups of living things. There are several characteristics that are common to all forms of life.

Characteristics

1) Organization The **cell** is the basic unit of all life. Any **organism** or living thing is a composition of cells. An organism can be **unicellular** (composed of only one cell) or **multi-cellular** (composed of more than one cell). Multi-cellular organisms begin life as a single cell. The organism grows as the single cell divides and the new cells undergo **differentiation**. That is, the cells take on the roles dictated by the genetic instructions within the cell.

2) Energy Use All organisms have the ability to maintain a very stable internal environment. This internal stability is called **homeostasis**. All organisms require energy to maintain homeostasis, to grow, and to reproduce. The process by which organisms use energy is called **metabolism**.

3) Reproduction Reproduction is another process common to all organisms. Scientifically speaking, this is the ability to produce a new organism that is like the original. This happens through transmission of hereditary information to the offspring in the form of deoxyribonucleic acid or DNA. DNA is a large molecule that contains information on development of certain traits for a particular organism. Traits are controlled by **genes**. While each cell in an organism contains information for all genes, each cell utilizes only the information needed to carry out its specific function. There are two types of reproduction, asexual and sexual. In **asexual reproduction**, only one parent is necessary to produce offspring. **Sexual reproduction** occurs when two parents are necessary to produce offspring.

4) Adaptation to the environment Over time, organisms have evolved (changed). Scientists suggest that this **evolution** has occurred through a process called **natural selection**. The theory states that those organisms with the most favorable traits are most successful in reproduction, thus making it more likely that the favorable traits will occur in the offspring.

5) Homeostasis Eukaryotes all have a membrane-bound nucleus, membrane-bound organelles, and a membrane surrounding the entire cell. This is, however, where the similarities stop. The nucleus and other organelles within the cell determine the functions for that cell. The cell membrane serves to protect the cell by allowing only some substances to pass through. The membrane is called selectively permeable because some substances can easily pass through and others cannot pass through at all. The cell membrane helps an organism maintain homeostasis by controlling what enters and leaves. The transport across the membrane is called **passive transport**. This movement will be discussed in more detail after a short review of chemistry.

The Cell

As already mentioned, the cell is the smallest unit of any life form that carries all the information needed for all life processes. Three things are true for all cells.

1. All living things consist of one or more cells. In multi-cellular organisms, the cells vary in size, shape, and internal organization.
2. Cells are the basic structures of any organism.
3. Cells can only reproduce from existing cells.

Cells work together in multi-cellular organisms to perform a function. The DNA in each cell contains the code necessary for the organism to combine proteins. Within a cell, there are structures called **organelles** that perform functions within the cell. Cells can be organized into groups based on one feature. There are those cells that have a **cell membrane** that not only surrounds the entire cell, but also surrounds the nucleus and other organelles. And, there are those cells in which the cell membrane does not surround the nucleus. Cells with a membrane around the nucleus are called **eukaryotes**, and those without are **prokaryotes**. Prokaryotes are unicellular organisms such as bacteria.

Think it Through

1. List three characteristics that all living things have in common.
2. Plant cells have a rigid structure that surrounds the entire cell outside of the cell membrane. Animal cells do not have this supportive and protective structure. Why do you think that animal cells do not have a cell wall?

Answers

1. All organisms reproduce, use energy through a process called metabolism, consist of cells, contain DNA, adapt to the environment, and maintain internal stability through homeostasis.
2. The purpose of the cell wall is to support and protect the plant. A rigid cell wall allows a plant to stand upright (in the case of bark on a tree) and/or be protected from a variety of pests. There are actually two types of cell wall. The primary cell wall allows for growth and flexibility while the plant matures. The secondary cell wall is tough as in the case of bark. A flexible cell wall allows more movement. Most animals contain cells with flexible cell walls and membranes for movement and cells with rigid cell walls for support.

Chemistry of the Cell

There are two types of cellular transport. Passive transport does not require the cell to expend any energy for movement of substances. Active transport, on the other hand, does require the cell to invest energy.

Passive Transport

The simplest form of passive transport is **diffusion**. Diffusion is the transfer of molecules from an area of high concentration to an area of lower concentration (down the concentration gradient). Concentration is the amount of solute (substance dissolved in solution) dissolved in a fixed amount of a solution. Diffusion uses only the **kinetic energy** (energy of motion) naturally found in a molecule. Molecules move constantly because of their kinetic energy. The movement tends to be in a straight line until the molecule bumps into something. When this happens, the molecule changes direction. Since higher concentrations in solutions mean there are more objects into which a molecule can collide, molecules tend to move down the concentration gradient from areas of high concentration to areas of lower concentration.

The process of water molecules moving down the concentration gradient is known as **osmosis**. If a solution is **hypotonic** (concentration outside is lower than inside) to the cell, then water moves into the cell to establish equilibrium. If a solution is **hypertonic** (concentration outside is higher than inside) to the cell, then water moves out of the cell to establish equilibrium. If the solution is **isotonic**, then water moves in and out of the cell because equilibrium has already been established. The presence of solute particles on either side of the membrane creates an osmotic pressure, which is proportional to the concentration, but independent of the type of particle.

Cells can be in an isotonic, hypotonic, or hypertonic environment. Cells in an isotonic external environment easily balance the movement of water across the cell membrane. This is typical of most vertebrates. Unicellular organisms in hypotonic environments continually move water in, but they have to remove this excess water. They have to expend energy to pump the water out (active transport). Similarly, multi-cellular organisms require active transport to remove water from the cell. Finally, some cells live in hypertonic environments. In these instances, water leaves the cell through osmosis.

Facilitated diffusion occurs when molecules cannot diffuse across a cell membrane even though there is a concentration gradient. The diffusion is facilitated by special proteins called **carrier proteins**. The carrier protein binds to a molecule on one side of the cell membrane. The protein changes shape in an effort to protect the molecule as it moves through the membrane. Once through the membrane, the molecule is released into the area of lower concentration.

Active Transport

If a cell must move up a concentration gradient, then energy is necessary. If this is the case, then active transport occurs.

Carrier proteins can serve in active transport as well. They tend to be called "pumps" because the proteins have to push the molecules from an area of lower concentration to an area of higher concentration. An example of such a protein is a sodium-potassium pump. This particular pump works to maintain proper concentrations of potassium and sodium in animal cells.

Two other types of active transport work to move large quantities of a substance into and out of cells at a single time. **Endocytosis** occurs when external substances are enclosed within the cell membrane and the pouch closes off and moves into the cell as a membrane-bound organelle. As its name suggests, **exocytosis** is essentially the opposite of endocytosis. The membrane-bound organelle fuses to the cell membrane and its contents are released external to the cell.

Think it Through

1. Distinguish between isotonic, hypotonic, and hypertonic solutions.
2. Describe the similarities and differences between active and passive transport.

Answers

1. An isotonic solution occurs when a solution is in equilibrium across a membrane. The solute concentration is lower outside the cell than within in a hypotonic environment. This means that water will diffuse into a cell. In a hypertonic environment, the solute concentration is higher outside the cell than within, and water diffuses out of the cell.
2. Active transport requires energy other than the kinetic energy found in molecules. Both active and passive transport allow movement of substances across a cell membrane.

Genetics

Genetics is the study of how traits are transported from parent to offspring, or heredity. Gregor Mendel began researching how characteristics of pea plants were passed to offspring from parent plants. He studied seven contrasting pairs of characteristics. He looked at plant height (long or short stems), flower position along stem (axial or terminal), pod appearance (inflated or constricted), pod color (green or yellow), seed color (green or yellow), flower color (purple or white), and seed texture (smooth or wrinkled). He collected seeds from various plants and recorded the characteristics of each plant. He planted the seeds the next year and noticed that it was possible for different traits to occur than those shown by the parent plant. Mendel went further than these first observations. He also cross-pollinated plants showing **pure** traits. A plant shows a pure trait if its offspring always have the same trait.

From his research, Mendel found that there are **dominant** and **recessive** traits. That is, he found that some traits always dominated the other in the first generation. Those traits that did not show up in this generation (recessive) only occurred in the second generation when both parents had the recessive trait. Recall that a gene is a section of DNA that controls a particular genetic trait on a chromosome. As presented here, there are multiple forms of a gene. These alternative forms are called **alleles**. Alleles are represented using letters. Dominant alleles get a capital letter, while recessive alleles are represented by a lowercase letter. The genotype (genetic makeup) of an organism consists of alleles inherited from both parents. The appearance of an organism resulting from its genotype is the phenotype. When both parents give the offspring the same allele, the offspring is **homozygous** for that particular trait. If the parents do not give the offspring the same allele for a particular trait, the offspring is **heterozygous** for that trait.

To predict what characteristics would occur in offspring, a Punnett square can be used. Below are some examples of various crosses.

Homozygous rose with thorns (T) x Homozygous rose without thorns (t)

	T	T
t	Tt	Tt
t	Tt	Tt

As you can see, all rose offspring will have thorns since one parent is homozygous for the dominant trait.

Homozygous rose with thorns (T) x Heterozygous rose with thorns (Tt)

	T	T
T	TT	TT
t	Tt	Tt

In this case, there is still no possibility of finding a rose without thorns among the offspring since one parent is homozygous for the dominant trait.

Heterozygous rose with thorns (Tt) x Homozygous rose without thorns (tt)

	T	t
t	Tt	tt
t	Tt	tt

Here, two of the offspring will have thorns, and two will not. That is, the offspring have a 50% chance of having thorns. Note that the only time the offspring will not have thorns is when they are homozygous for the recessive trait.

Heterozygous rose with thorns (Tt) x Heterozygous rose with thorns (Tt)

	T	t
T	TT	Tt
t	Tt	tt

When two heterozygous plants are crossed, two of the offspring will be homozygous. One will be homozygous for the dominant trait and one will be homozygous for the recessive trait. The other two offspring will be heterozygous. Of course, another way of looking at this is that 75% of the offspring will have thorns and 25% will not.

Think it Through

1. An offspring can be homozygous for the dominant trait or heterozygous and show the dominant trait. How could you determine if the parents are heterozygous or homozygous?
2. Based on your knowledge of genetics and this brief review, what does incomplete dominance mean?

Answers

1. Try crossing each parent with a known homozygous recessive individual. If you cross a heterozygous dominant with a homozygous recessive, then 50% of the offspring will be homozygous recessive and 50% will be heterozygous. This is called a **testcross**.
2. Think about red and white carnations. If one color was dominant and the other completely recessive, then there would be no pink carnations. Incomplete dominance occurs when the alleles each influence the trait in the offspring with neither necessarily dominating the other. The resulting phenotype is intermediate between two parents.

Test Information

The examination you are about to take is multiple choice with only one correct answer per item. Photocopy the answer sheet on this page to record your choices. Circle the correct answer on your answer sheet for each test item. When you have completed the practice test, you may check your answers with those listed on the answer key that follows the Life Science Practice Test questions.

Life Science Practice Test
Answer Sheet

1.	a	b	c	d	24.	a	b	c	d
2.	a	b	c	d	25.	a	b	c	d
3.	a	b	c	d	26.	a	b	c	d
4.	a	b	c	d	27.	a	b	c	d
5.	a	b	c	d	28.	a	b	c	d
6.	a	b	c	d	29.	a	b	c	d
7.	a	b	c	d	30.	a	b	c	d
8.	a	b	c	d	31.	a	b	c	d
9.	a	b	c	d	32.	a	b	c	d
10.	a	b	c	d	33.	a	b	c	d
11.	a	b	c	d	34.	a	b	c	d
12.	a	b	c	d	35.	a	b	c	d
13.	a	b	c	d	36.	a	b	c	d
14.	a	b	c	d	37.	a	b	c	d
15.	a	b	c	d	38.	a	b	c	d
16.	a	b	c	d	39.	a	b	c	d
17.	a	b	c	d	40.	a	b	c	d
18.	a	b	c	d	41.	a	b	c	d
19.	a	b	c	d	42.	a	b	c	d
20.	a	b	c	d	43.	a	b	c	d
21.	a	b	c	d	44.	a	b	c	d
22.	a	b	c	d	45.	a	b	c	d
23.	a	b	c	d	46.	a	b	c	d

Questions 1-2 relate to the concepts of osmosis and diffusion, as shown in the following diagram.

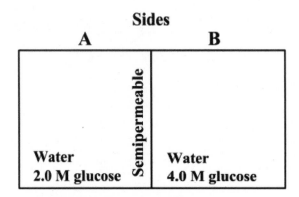

Sides

A   **B**

Water
2.0 M glucose

Semipermeable

Water
4.0 M glucose

**Diffusion-Osmosis:
Two Solutions of Glucose Separated
by a Semipermeable Membrane.**

1. At the initial concentrations, side B relative to A, is:
    a. hypertonic
    b. lower
    c. isotonic
    d. hypotonic

2. Which molecule moves across the membrane in order to reach equilibrium?
    a. water only
    b. glucose and water
    c. glucose only
    d. nothing will move

In humans, the hypothetical disease Allomentia, is carried on the allele "a," which is recessive to "A" for the normal condition. **Use the Punnett squares in the following diagrams to answer questions 3, 4, and 5.**

Figure 1

	A	A
a	Aa	Aa
a	Aa	Aa

F_1

Figure 2

	A	a
A	AA	Aa
a	Aa	aa

F_2

3. A normal (AA) male is mated with an allomentic (aa) female. What is the percentage of offspring in the F_1 generation (first generation after crossing two parental lines) with the disease?
   a. 100%
   b. 75%
   c. 25%
   d. 0%

4. The percentage of F_2 offspring (generation produced from F_1 generation) that are carriers of allomentia is:
   a. 0%.
   b. 25%.
   c. 50%.
   d. 75%.

5. The allele frequency of A and a in the F_2 generation is:
   a. 0.5:A and 0.25:a.
   b. 0.25:A and 0.5:a.
   c. 0.25:A and 0.25:a.
   d. 0.5:A and 0.5:a.

Phenotype characteristics that are carried by genes on X chromosomes are termed **sex-linked**. Sex-linked traits are recessive to normal X chromosomes but not to Y chromosomes. **Use the following diagram to answer questions 6 through 9.**

6. When a normal (XY) male mates with a color-blind (xx) female, the percentage of color-blind children (male:female) in the F_1 generation will be:
   a. 0 male:100 female.
   b. 50 male:50 female.
   c. 100 male:100 female.
   d. 100 male:0 female.

	Y	X
x	Yx	Xx
x	Yx	Xx

F_1

Monohybrid Cross of a Normal and a Sex-Linked Disease Individual

7. Color-blindness is a recessive trait found on the X chromosome. If a color-blind mother mates with a normal father, the mother can give birth to:
    a. only color-blind boys and normal girls.
    b. one-half carrier boys and one-half carrier girls.
    c. only carrier girls and color-blind boys.
    d. only normal boys and color-blind girls.

A DNA molecule is composed of two helical chains that contain the bases adenine, thymine, cytosine, and guanine (A, T, C, G), respectively. The two chains are held together by mandated base pairing of A to T and C to G.

```
Chain I      A A T ——— C G C ——— T A T ——— G C G
             | | |      | | |      | | |      | | |
Chain II     T T A ——— G C G ——— A T A ——— C G C
```

Sections of a DNA molecule form genes which direct the synthesis of structural and functional proteins. The DNA molecules unzip and serve as a blueprint for making DNA and RNA. The genetic message of DNA is transcribed into mRNA (messenger RNA) and is translated by tRNA (transfer RNA) to establish the proper amino acid sequence. Instead of thymine as in DNA, RNA contains the base uracil (U) that pairs with adenine. This is one difference between DNA and RNA. Another difference is that the sugar in DNA is deoxyribose. In RNA, the sugar is called ribose. Chain I (above) is the blueprint that was used to generate the mRNA below. **Use the description below to answer questions 8 and 9.**

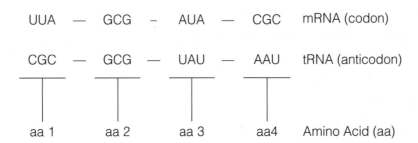

8. Translate the mRNA (codon) from left to right by selecting the proper amino acid sequence to create the corresponding tRNA (anticodon).
    a. 2-1-4-3
    b. 3-1-2-4
    c. 4-1-3-2
    d. 1-2-3-4

9. Which statement is correct?
    a. Thymine pairs with adenine in RNA.
    b. Cytosine replaces thymine in tRNA.
    c. DNA contains the sugar ribose.
    d. RNA contains the sugar ribose.

10. If the alleles of the parents are known, how does a Punnett square help in predicting the genotype of the offspring?
    a. provides probabilities of getting an incomplete dominance
    b. shows exactly what genotypes will occur in the offspring
    c. provides information on dominant traits in the parents
    d. shows what parents would be the best to cross to encourage a trait

Scientific research generally involves the collection of data from laboratory, clinical or field experiments, or observations. The data represent samples of specific parameters that exist in nature. The larger the sample size (n), the closer its values approximate the value of the entire population in question. Just as one measure of reliable data is its reproducibility, a scientist should not draw conclusions from a single count or measurement. Numerous replications of data are required to increase the confidence level.

Questions 11 through 26 are designed to review your comprehension of scientific reasoning.

A 10 ml volume of distilled H_2O with a pinch of *serratia marcescens* bacteria was serially diluted in order to do a cell count of the sample. **Use the figure to answer questions 11 and 12.**

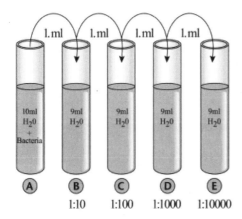

Serial Dilution of a 10.0 ml Volume
of Bacterial Cells

11. In <u>each</u> dilution from tube B to tube E, the number of bacteria/ml is reduced by:
    a. 9/10
    b. 10/10
    c. 2/10
    d. 1/10

12. If the number of cells in tube D is 500/ml, the number in tube B was:
    a. 45,000.
    b. 50,000.
    c. 5,500.
    d. 5,000.

The growth in bacterial colonies is consistent with simple mathematical expressions for population dynamics and is expressed quantitatively as:

Growth(G) = $\dfrac{\Delta N}{\Delta t}$ (Change in population size)
(Change in time)

Cell counts taken from bacterial colonies were plotted as a function of time. **Use the following diagram to answer questions 13 and 14.**

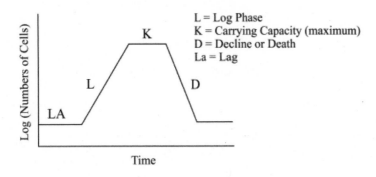

13. At position K on the bacterial growth curve, the expression $\Delta N / \Delta t$ is close to:
    a. 100.
    b. 1.0.
    c. 50.0.
    d. 0.0.

14. Choose the correct statement.
    a. Maximum growth occurs at K.
    b. Low growth occurs at D.
    c. Maximum $\dfrac{\Delta N}{\Delta t}$ occurs at L.
    d. Minimum growth occurs at L.

Nonscientists mistakenly assume that **accuracy** and **precision** are synonymous, but it is important for scientists to understand the differences between them.

Accuracy is the degree of <u>correctness</u> of a measurement and precision is its <u>level of reproducibility</u>. The data in each of the following samples represent 10 separate measurements of the mass (kg) of cattle.

Sample 1—   25 – 30 – 35 – 40 – 50 – 50 – 60 – 70 – 80 – 85
Sample 2—   20 – 20 – 22 – 20 – 21 – 19 – 19 – 19 – 21 – 20

If the mean mass of the cattle is 50 kg, which statement is best supported by the data for Samples 1 and 2, respectively?

15.   Sample 1:
       a.   low accuracy and high precision
       b.   high accuracy and low precision
       c.   low precision and low accuracy
       d.   high precision and high accuracy

16.   Sample 2:
       a.   low precision and low accuracy
       b.   high precision and high accuracy
       c.   high accuracy and low precision
       d.   high precision and low accuracy

17.   How should a researcher test the hypothesis that soy is a superior diet to whole wheat for the reproduction of flour beetles, *Tribolium confusum*?
       a.   Record the number of eggs recovered from a single culture reared on soy versus on whole wheat.
       b.   Count the eggs recovered from 10 separate cultures reared on soy versus a single culture on whole wheat.
       c.   Compare the eggs from 10 soy cultures versus 10 whole wheat cultures.
       d.   Record the eggs from one soy culture versus 10 whole wheat cultures.

18.   The best clinical protocol to test the hypothesis that good cholesterol (HDL) flushes out bad cholesterol (LDL) from the arteries of humans is to treat:
       a.   one patient with a single dosage of HDL medication, followed by periodic blood tests.
       b.   six groups (10 patient/group), with the same dosage of HDL medication, followed by a single blood test.
       c.   six groups (10 patients/group), with each group receiving a different dosage of HDL, followed by periodic blood tests.
       d.   one group of 10 patients, with each person receiving a different dosage of HDL, followed by periodic blood tests.

A flour beetle, *Tribolium confusum*, culture was started with 10 males and 10 females in a 20 mL flask. The diet consisted of whole wheat flour. The population increased to 940 insects, after which the number remained constant for several days, followed by an increase in the death rate.

19. The hypothesis being tested by the beetle experiment was:
    a. the population is controlled by density-dependent factors.
    b. the insects can reproduce on whole wheat.
    c. the population is controlled by density-independent factors.
    d. death rate is indirectly proportional to density.

20. When two closely related species of flour beetles, *T. confusum* and *T. castaneum* were placed in culture in equal numbers, *T. castaneum* increased in numbers while *T. confusum* experienced population decline. The population growth differences most likely indicate that the energy consumption efficiency of *T. confusum* in relation to *T. castaneum* is:
    a. *T. confusum* > *T. castaneum*.
    b. equal in the two species.
    c. *T. castaneum* > *T. confusum*.
    d. not reflected by the data.

21. A research student was given the assignment to determine the pollen count for a 24-hour period in a given location. His data would be most reliable if he decided to count pollen in:
    a. a single decimeter square for one morning and one afternoon.
    b. multiple decimeter squares for one morning and one afternoon.
    c. a single decimeter square for one afternoon.
    d. multiple decimeter squares for one afternoon.

Francesco Redi's experiments refuted the spontaneous generation of maggots in meat. When meat is exposed in an open jar, flies lay their eggs on it, and the eggs hatch into maggots (fly larvae). In a sealed jar, however, no maggots appear. If the jar is covered with gauze, maggots hatch from eggs that the flies lay on top of the gauze, but still no maggots appear in the meat. **Use the diagram to answer question 22.**

22. Which of the jars in Redi's experiment served best to refute spontaneous generation?
    a. the first jar
    b. the second jar
    c. the third jar
    d. none

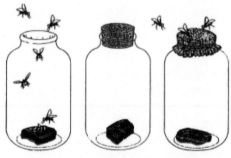

Francesco Redi's Experiment
Refutation of the Spontaneous
Generation of Maggots on Meat
(After: Black, 1996)

Use the following information to answer questions 23 and 24.

Robert Koch (1843-1910), a German physician, helped to establish the Germ Theory of Infectious Disease by a chain of postulates that bear his name. The postulates demonstrated that a specific pathogen was capable of generating disease in a human host. Koch's Postulates entailed: (1) recovering a suspected pathogen from a disease host, (2) growing the pathogen on a culture medium, (3) isolating the pathogen, (4) establishing the pathogen's identity.

23. What is the most logical step (5) of the postulate?
    a. Inject the isolated pathogen into a diseased host to determine if its condition worsens.
    b. Inject the isolated pathogen into a healthy host and monitor for signs and symptoms of disease.
    c. Serially dilute the pathogen and see if it will continue to grow in pure culture.
    d. None of the above.

24. Pathogenic bacteria stimulate the release of macrophages which release interleukins that activate prostaglandins. This causes a rise in body temperature (fever). The best experimental protocol based on Koch's theory is to test the hypothesis that acetyl salicylic acid (aspirin) reduces fever is to treat:
    a. one patient with 6×10^2 mg aspirin. Take his/her temperature initially and every hour for six hours.
    b. six patients with 6×10^2 mg aspirin and follow the same protocol as in option a.
    c. six patients with 6×10^2 mg aspirin and check their temperatures in 5 minutes.
    d. six patients and check their temperatures in 24 hours.

The following section contains reasoning problems associated with biological relationships. Questions 25 through 28 use modified Venn diagrams to express evolutionary diversity among selected vertebrate and invertebrate species. Note the specific independence and overlap of geometric figures that express these associations. **Use the following diagram to answer question 25.**

25. Choose the statement most consistent with this overlap of geometric diagrams.
    a. A spider is an insect, an arthropod, and an orthopteran.
    b. A cricket is an arthropod, an insect, and an orthopteran.
    c. A beetle is an arthropod, an insect, and an orthopteran.
    d. A butterfly is an orthopteran, an insect, and an arthropod.

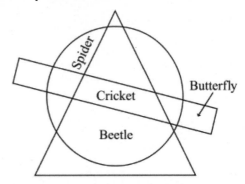

Overlap of Geometric Figures,
Relating Taxonomic Categories
(Circle-Arthropods, Triangle-Insects,
and Rectangle-Orthopterans)

Use the diagram to the right to answer questions 26 and 27.

26. Choose the correct statement, consistent with the diagram. A cat is:
    a. an ungulate, a mammal, and a vertebrate.
    b. a vertebrate and an ungulate.
    c. a mammal and a vertebrate.
    d. a mammal only.

27. According to the diagram, a horse is:
    a. a vertebrate and an ungulate, but not a mammal.
    b. a mammal, but not an ungulate.
    c. a mammal and an ungulate, but not a vertebrate.
    d. an ungulate, a mammal and a vertebrate.

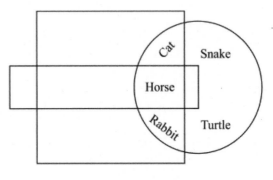

Overlap of Geometric Figures,
Relating Taxonomic Categories
(Circle-Vertebrates, Square Mammals,
and Rectangle-Ungulates)

Use the following diagram to answer question 28.

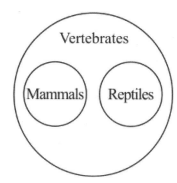

Venn Diagram Showing
Two Classes of Vertebrates

28. The correct statement expressed by the Venn diagram is:
   a. All mammals are vertebrates, but not all mammals are reptiles.
   b. All mammals are vertebrates, but not all vertebrates are mammals.
   c. Some reptiles are mammals, but no mammals are reptiles.
   d. No reptiles are vertebrates.

A survivorship curve depicts the number or the percentage of offspring alive throughout the life span of the species. **Use the following diagram to answer questions 29 and 30.**

29. The human species conforms to which of these survival types?
   a. T1
   b. T2
   c. T3
   d. T1 and T2

30. The highest mortality is shortly after birth in:
   a. T3
   b. T2
   c. T1
   d. There is no way to determine this.

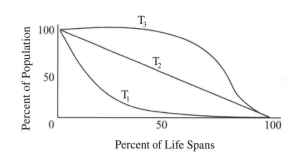

Survivorship Curves Showing
Three Types of Life Patterns

The trophic levels or food chain in an ecosystem can be used to construct pyramids of energy flow. Radiant energy from the sun enters an ecosystem when PRODUCERS (green plants) use it to produce food molecules which are eaten by PRIMARY, SECONDARY and TERTIARY CONSUMERS (e.g. herbivores, carnivores, and second-level carnivores, respectively). Animals, plants and microbes in all ecosystems also form pyramids of numbers, biomass, and energy.

According to The Second Law of Thermodynamics, the efficiency of energy transfer between levels of an energy pyramid is always < 1.0, with varying quantities of energy released as heat. **Use the following diagram to answer questions 31 through 34.**

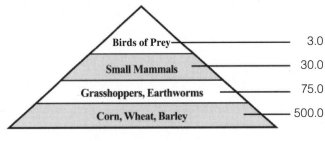

Ecosystem Pyramids of Numbers,
Biomass, and Energy

In elementary physics, efficiency is defined as the ratio of energy output per energy input.

Efficiency = Output/Input x 100

Gross primary productivity (GPP) is the total amount of radiant energy converted to chemical energy by green plants in a given area per unit of time.

31. The following are statements about the energy efficiency in nutrient consumption. Which statement is correct?
    a. Birds of Prey > Grasshoppers and Earthworms
    b. Small Mammals = Grasshoppers and Earthworms
    c. Birds of Prey > Small Mammals
    d. Grasshoppers and Earthworms > Birds of Prey

32. Choose the correct statement regarding Energy Content (Kcals/Kg – Biomass).
    a. Small Mammals > Grasshoppers and Earthworms
    b. Birds of Prey = Small Mammals
    c. Grasshoppers and Earthworms > Small Mammals
    d. Birds of Prey > Grasshopper and Earthworms

33. Of the 30,000 calories of potential energy fixed during photosynthesis by corn, wheat, and barley, the efficiency of energy harvest was 60%. Using the equation above, the original number of calories absorbed from the sun was:
    a. 50,000.
    b. 60,000.
    c. 5,000.
    d. 6,000.

34. The efficiency of energy of primary productivity is greater if one eats:
    a. vegetables.
    b. combination (meat and vegetables).
    c. meat.
    d. his/her personal choice.

As sunlight strikes the leaves of plants, its individual colors must be absorbed to promote photosynthesis. Portions of the light that are not absorbed are reflected to the human eyes as colors. **Use the following diagram to answer questions 35 and 36.**

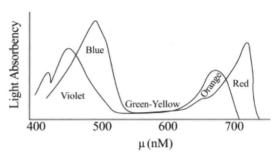

Absorption Spectra of Sunlight (400nM-750nM)

35. From the absorption spectrum, choose the two colors least effective in promoting photosynthesis.
    a.   blue/green
    b.   red/blue
    c.   orange/green
    d.   green/yellow

36. The light absorption spectrum in the figure indicates that the most efficient wavelength pattern for photosynthesis is:
    a.   long wavelength – low absorption.
    b.   short wavelength – low absorption.
    c.   short wavelength – high absorption.
    d.   long wavelength – high absorption.

Use the following diagram to answer questions 37 through 39.

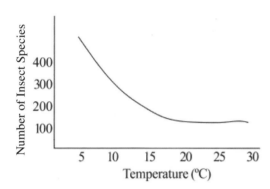

Species Diversity as a Function of Increasing Temperature (0°C)

37. The correlation between species diversity and temperature is:
    a.   direct.
    b.   scattered.
    c.   inverse.
    d.   non-existent.

38. The graph suggests that the largest number of species are adapted:
    a.   to cold temperatures near 5°.
    b.   equally to cold and warm temperatures.
    c.   to warm temperatures near 30°.
    d.   to temperatures near 15°.

39. A certain type of insect is developed in a climate-controlled lab. The insect population is 5,000 at a temperature of 20°C and 2,000 at a temperature of 25°C. An electrical outage in the lab disengages the climate control system. Based on the graph, what should happen to the insect population at a temperature of 10°C? (Assume that this insect population is typical of those shown in the graph.)
    a.   The population will decrease.
    b.   The population will increase.
    c.   The population will stay the same.
    d.   There is not enough information to answer.

In proportionality relationships, two variables are directly proportional when their ratio is a constant, EqA (K = y/x). When their product is a constant, the variables are inversely proportional, EqB (K = XY). To **interpolate** is to estimate values between two known values.

Use this diagram to answer questions 40 through 42.

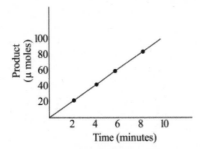

Enzyme Activity as a
Function of Time (minutes)

40. In the enzyme-catalyzed reaction where μ moles of product are produced over time, the data support:
    a. Eq B.
    b. both Eq A and Eq B.
    c. Eq A.
    d. neither Eq.

41. The value of the implied constant (K) is:
    a. 40.
    b. 20.
    c. 1.
    d. 10.

42. The value of y when x equals 10 is:
    a. 90.
    b. 120.
    c. 85.
    d. not able to be interpolated from the standard curve.

Use the following diagram to answer questions 43 through 46.

43. The cricket died from a microsporidia disease; subsequently, the eagle became infected by:
    a. primary meal of squirrel.
    b. secondary meal of shrew.
    c. secondary meal of lizard.
    d. primary meal of wheat.

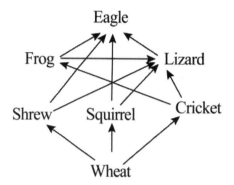

44. It is known that chlorinated hydrocarbon pesticides are biological concentrators (built up along trophic levels). Choose the correct relationship relative to long-term concentration of pesticide after the wheat is treated for insects.
    a. Lizard > Cricket
    b. Shrew ≈ Lizard
    c. Shrew > Eagle
    d. Lizard > Eagle

45. In relation to the provided ecosystem, which statement is correct?
    a. The energy content in squirrels is lower than that in eagles.
    b. Frogs and lizards occupy the second trophic level.
    c. The energy content in wheat is higher than that in frogs.
    d. Eagles occupy the first trophic level.

46. Drought conditions lowered the wheat crop by one-third in a certain year. What effect would this decline in wheat have on the rest of the ecosystem?
    a. The shrew, squirrel, and cricket would occupy the first trophic level, but nothing else would change.
    b. The squirrel population would decline, but the population of shrews and crickets would not.
    c. The lizard population would decline, but nothing else would change.
    d. All populations would decline since there would be a wheat shortage.

END OF THE TEST

Life Science Practice Test Answer Key

1.   a   There is a higher concentration of glucose on side B. To reach equilibrium, water will move from side A to side B. Thus, initially side B is hypertonic to side A.

2.   a   Glucose does not diffuse across a semi-permeable membrane. However, the smaller water molecules will diffuse across the membrane by osmosis from side A to side B until both sides are isotonic.

3.   d   The disease, Allomentia, is carried on the gene "a" which occurs in all progeny of the F_1 generation in a heterozygous Aa state. This dominant gene "A" will suppress phenotypic expression of the disease in the entire generation.

4.   c   The Punnett square in Figure 2 shows that two of the four F_2 offspring are heterozygous (Aa) with one gene for the disease.

5.   d   Note that each box of the Punnett square in Figures 1 and 2 represents 25 percent of the generation. When the percentage is converted to a decimal and the square root extracted, the individual gene frequency is derived (e.g., 25% = 0.25 = 0.5). Also, the allele frequency can be determined by counting the number of each allele (A,a) and dividing the total to determine the proportion.

6.   d   All the F1 males are color-blind because the gene carried on the X chromosome is not recessive to the Y. This gene is recessive to the X in females, which makes all F_1 females carriers.

7.   c   Because females possess 2 X chromosomes with one dominant to sex-linked genes, a color-blind mother can only produce carrier daughters and color-blind sons when the father is normal.

8.   c   The base pairing on the mRNA must be compatibly matched with those of the tRNA as follows:

                    U U A   G C G   A U A   C G C
                    A A U   C G C   U A U   G C G
                     4   1   3   2

9.   d   The DNA molecule contains a ribose sugar that is lacking an oxygen atom. The sugar is deoxyribose. RNA contains the sugar ribose.

10.   d   A trait can be encouraged or discouraged based on the probabilities found when crossing two parents to create offspring.

11.   a   Each time a 1.0 ml aliquot is put into enough solvent to equal a 10 ml final volume, the solution is diluted by 9/10.

12.   b   The cell count in each vial is 0.1 the count in the preceding vial (e.g., vial D = 500, vial C = 5,000, and vial B = 50,000).

13.   d   Position K (carrying capacity) is the point of which a bacterial population has made maximum use of nutrients and has reached a point at which the environment cannot support any additional increase in numbers. Therefore, there is no further change in numbers (ΔN) per change in time (Δt).

14.   c   At position L, the growth curve has a maximum positive slope indicating maximum increase in number (ΔN) per change in time (Δt).

15.   b   Sample 1 of the measurements representing cattle weights have a wide range, but they are clumped around the mean value of the actual weight.

16. d   In Sample 2, the measurements representing cattle weights are clumped within a narrow range, but are significantly removed from the actual weight indicating a greater precision of measurement, but low accuracy.

17. c   The protocol in option c gives enough replicates on each diet to determine the accuracy and precision of the experiment and increase the statistical significance of the data.

18. c   The protocol in option c gives the same advantages as in the previous question. An additional advantage is that because humans are the experimental subjects, there is opportunity to observe an individual patient's responses to the drugs.

19. a   In the absence of a K factor (carrying capacity), which limited population increase to 940 insects, growth would have continued exponentially, independent of population density.

20. c   Nutrition is necessary for growth in all animals. Therefore, growth is positively correlated with utilization of nutrients.

21. b   Counts in several squares provide a sufficient sample size and counts from morning and afternoon indicate the pollen distribution throughout the day.

22. c   Jar 3 in the experiment demonstrated that when the flies were prevented from contacting the meat, no maggots developed on it; proving that decaying meat does not become maggots. The maggots developed from fly eggs deposited on top of the gauze.

23. b   The injection of a pathogen from a pure culture tests the hypothesis that it is the causative agent of the disease in question.

24. b   The protocol in option b affords replicates (numbers of patients and numbers of temperature readings) that measure the accuracy and the reproducibility of a clinical investigation.

25. b   Option b is the most consistent description with the geometric pattern, because a cricket belongs to the phylum of arthropoda, the class of insects, and the order of orthoptera.

26. c   Option c illustrates that a cat is a vertebrate and a mammal because it occupies the circle and the square.

27. d   Option d demonstrates that because a horse occupies the rectangle, the square and the circle, it is an ungulate mammalian vertebrate.

28. b   The vertebrates represent a subphylum that contains both mammals and reptiles. The small circles are inside the large circle but do not overlap.

29. c   The curve in option c shows that in humans, most individuals survive until the last part of the mean life span.

30. c   The curve in option c shows high mortality among young individuals of the T_1 group.

31. d   The energy efficiency in grasshoppers and earthworms exceeds that in birds of prey because the former are herbivores that occupy the second trophic level, and the latter are secondary carnivores that occupy a higher trophic level.

32. c   The energy content in grasshoppers and earthworms is greater than that in small mammals because they occupy a lower level of an upright pyramid of energy.

33. a   The energy absorbed from the sun was determined by rearranging the formula to solve for energy input
$$\text{(e.g., } E = OP/IP \ (100) \text{ to: } IP = OP \ (100)/E)$$

34.   a   Energy efficiency is greater if one eats vegetables because vegetables are producers, and producers have a higher energy efficiency than other levels of the biomass pyramid.

35.   d   Green and yellow are the least absorbed colors in the visual portion of the spectrum. Color must be absorbed to promote photosynthesis, hence plants typically appear green and yellow.

36.   c   The violet and blue portions of the visible spectrum are the most efficient at promoting photosynthesis. They have the shortest wavelength (400 nm).

37.   c   The curve indicates that as temperature increases, the number of species decreases.

38.   a   The curve shows that most species are better adapted to cold temperatures.

39.   b   Just as indicated in a previous question, the curve shows that populations decrease as temperature increases, so the inverse should also be true. That is, the population is higher at a lower temperature.

40.   c   Equation A, in which the ratio (Y/X) of the variables is a constant (K) is consistent with the graph which shows a straight line slope.

41.   d   The data show that each Y value divided by its corresponding X value equals the constant K value of 10.

42.   d   The value cannot be interpolated from the graph because interpolations must be made between two known points.

43.   c   The trophic relationship of the ecosystem in the figure is such that eagles are birds of prey on smaller reptiles, such as lizards.

44.   a.   The hydrocarbon pesticides consumed by insects would accumulate in their tissues of any animal that uses them as prey. Since a lizard is on a higher trophic level and preys on insects, its pesticide concentration would be higher.

45.   c   The energy content is highest in the lowest levels of the ecosystem since energy enters any ecosystem from the sun.

46.   d   The occupants of the second trophic level would have less to eat. Thus, those populations would decline. Then, the frogs and lizards would have less to eat causing those populations to decline. Finally, the eagle population would decline since there would be fewer frogs, lizards and squirrels.

Human Body Science

Humans are clearly multi-cellular organisms. One cell divides and multiplies in such a way that the cellular groups that form can perform specific functions as dictated by the DNA codes within the cells. As you may recall from a few pages ago, DNA specifies how proteins will be combined. As the cells divide to form a human, an exact copy of the DNA material is passed on to the new cell. In this way, each cell within a person contains the same information.

Human body science can be divided into two subjects: **anatomy** and **physiology**. These areas describe how the human body functions. Anatomy is the study of the structure and shape of the body. Physiology is the study of how parts of the body function. Clearly, these two areas of human science are dependent on one another. For example, the structure of a particular body part indicates the function for that particular part.

Human Body Structure

The human body has a very complex structure. Atoms combine to form molecules. Specific molecules combine to form cells. Recall that individual cells vary in size, shape and function. Cells collect in terms of function and type to form **tissues**. There are four basic tissue types in humans. Two or more tissue types that work together to perform a specific function form an **organ**. At the organ level, it is possible to perform extremely complex functions. When organs work together to perform a task, then the result is an **organ system**. There are 11 organ systems in the human body. The highest level of organization is the **organism**. This is the result of the work of all organ systems within the body.

As previously mentioned, there are four basic tissue types in humans: epithelial, connective, nervous, and muscular tissues.

Epithelium serves two functions. The epithelial tissue can serve as covering (such as skin tissue) or as glandular tissue. Epithelial tissue has some common characteristics. This type of tissue connects in sheets. It does not have its own blood supply. So, epithelium is dependent on diffusion from the nearby capillaries for food and oxygen. Epithelial tissue can regenerate easily if well nourished. There are two major types of epithelium. The **simple epithelium** is one layer of cells. The simple type is used for absorption, secretion, and filtration. Clearly, one layer of cells does not provide much protection. **Stratified epithelium** has more than one layer of cells. As such, it is the stratified epithelial tissue that serves as protection.

Connective tissue is found throughout the body. It serves, as you might guess, to connect different parts of the body. A trait common to most connective tissue is that it has its own blood supply. However, there are some types, such as ligaments, that do not. Some types of connective tissue include bone, cartilage, adipose (fat) tissue, and blood (vascular) tissue.

Muscle tissue is dedicated to producing movement. There are several types of muscle tissue including skeletal, cardiac, and smooth muscle. **Skeletal** muscle allows for voluntary movement since it connects to the skeletal system. That is, movement is consciously controlled. **Smooth** muscle is under involuntary control. It is found in the walls of internal organs. Like smooth muscle, **cardiac** muscle movement is involuntary. Cardiac muscle is found only in the heart.

The last type of tissue is **nervous tissue**. This type of tissue makes up neurons. **Neurons** send electrical impulses throughout the body. Along with special cells that protect the nervous tissue (called supporting cells), the neurons make up the nervous system structures such as the brain, spinal cord, and nerves.

Organ Systems

There are 11 organ systems in the human body. The purpose of each, along with the organs included, will be discussed.

Integumentary system The integumentary system is the skin. It protects internal tissues from injury, waterproofs the body, and helps regulate body temperature. This system also serves as a barrier to foreign substances.

Skeletal system The skeletal system provides support and protection for the body and supplies a framework that muscle tissue uses to create movement. The skeletal system also serves as storage for minerals. It consists of bones, cartilage, ligaments, and joints.

Muscular system Recall from the short discussion on muscle tissue that muscles have only one purpose and that is to produce movement through contraction. The muscular system consists only of the skeletal muscles. The cardiac and smooth muscles are not included in this organ system.

Nervous system The nervous system consists of the brain, spinal cord, nerves, and sensory receptors, and serves as the body's control system. Sensory receptors in the nervous system detect stimuli that can occur both within and outside the body. Once stimuli are detected, the nervous system activates the appropriate muscles or glands to respond. The nervous system is very fast-acting since immediate response is necessary to protect the body from changes in the internal and external environment.

Endocrine system While the endocrine system also serves to control bodily functions, it works much more slowly than the nervous system. Glands in the endocrine system secrete hormones that travel through the blood to organs throughout the body. Glands such as the pineal, pituitary, thyroid, thymus, and adrenal regulate processes such as growth and metabolism. Also included in the endocrine system are the pancreas, testes, and ovaries.

Cardiovascular system The cardiac system consists of the heart, blood vessels, and blood. This system works as the travel system for many substances necessary for the body. Oxygen, hormones, and nutrients travel throughout the body in the blood.

Lymphatic system The lymphatic system consists of lymphatic nodes and vessels, the spleen, and thoracic duct. Its purpose is to return fluid that has leaked from the cardiovascular system to the blood vessels. This system helps cleanse the blood and houses the white blood cells that are involved in protecting the body from environmental factors. Thus, the work of the lymphatic system is very closely tied to the work of the cardiovascular system.

Respiratory system The respiratory system has two main jobs. It must keep all the cells in the body supplied with oxygen and remove the carbon dioxide. This system consists of the nasal cavity, pharynx, larynx, trachea, bronchi, and the lungs. The lungs house tiny air sacs called alveoli. It is through the walls of the alveoli that oxygen and carbon dioxide move in and out of blood vessels.

Digestive system The digestive system consists of all the organs from the mouth to the anus involved in processing food. The organs along the path include the esophagus, stomach, small and large intestines, and the rectum. The digestive system breaks down food so that the nutrients can be easily passed to the blood for circulation through the body. Any food that is not digested and utilized for cells in the body is expelled through the anus. The breakdown of the food actually ends in the small intestine. After that, the digestive system tries to remove water from the excess. Two other organs included in the digestive system include the liver and pancreas. The liver produces bile that helps break down fats, and the pancreas delivers enzymes to the small intestine.

Urinary system The urinary, or excretory, system helps maintain the water and salt balances within the body, regulates the acid-base balance in the blood, and removes all nitrogen-containing wastes from the body. The nitrogen-containing wastes are by-products of the breakdown of proteins and nucleic acids.

Reproductive system The main purpose of the reproductive system is to produce offspring. This system is specialized in men to produce sperm, and in women to produce eggs (or ova). The reproductive organs also house certain hormones that encourage or suppress activities within the body (e.g., aggression, masculine or feminine skeletal form).

Think it Through

1. What type of muscle tissue would you find in the digestive system?
2. Order the six levels of structural organization from most to least complex.

Answers

1. The digestive system consists of the organs that connect the mouth to the anus. These organs are surrounded by smooth muscle.
2. Note: MOST to LEAST
   Organismal, systemic, organ, tissue, cellular, chemical

Human Body Science Vocabulary

All individuals are derived from a single cell which multiplies to form distinct patterns or groupings of cells called tissues. Tissues grow and mature to form specific organs, and organs develop into systems which carry out the bodily functions. So, the human body is an integrated structure designed to carry out the functions of life. These functions include:

Adaptation— receive, interpret, and respond to internal and external stimuli via the nervous system

Circulation— transport oxygen and other nutrients to the tissues via the cardiovascular system

Elimination— remove metabolic wastes from the body via the renal system

Locomotion— voluntary and involuntary movement of body via the musculoskeletal system

Nutrition— take in and break down nutrients to be used for metabolism via the digestive system

Oxygenation— take in oxygen and expel carbon dioxide via the respiratory system

Regulation— hormonal control of bodily function via the endocrine system

Self-duplication— production of offspring via the reproductive system

Some Anatomical Terms

There are specific terms used in discussing anatomy that might be useful for you to review. They appear below. These terms and definitions will also be utilized in the practice test.

Anatomical position – a standard position in which the body is facing forward, feet are parallel, and the arms are at the sides with palms facing forward

Superior – toward the upper end of the body

Inferior – toward the lower end of the body (opposite of superior)

Anterior – toward the front of the body

Posterior – toward the back of the body (opposite of anterior)

Medial – toward the middle of the body

Lateral – toward the outer side of the body (opposite of medial)

Intermediate – between medial and lateral

Proximal – close to the trunk of the body

Distal – away from the trunk of the body (opposite of proximal)

Superficial – toward or at the body surface

Deep – away from the body surface (opposite of superficial)

Sagittal section – cut made along a longitudinal plane dividing the body into right and left parts

Midsagittal section – sagittal section made down the median of the body

Transverse section (cross section) – cut made along a horizontal plane to divide the body into upper and lower regions

Frontal section (coronal section) – cut made along a longitudinal plane that divides the body into front and back regions

Dorsal body cavity – contains the cranial cavity and spinal column

Ventral body cavity – contains all the structures within the chest and abdomen. The diaphragm divides the ventral cavity into the thoracic cavity (superior to the diaphragm) and the abdominal and pelvic cavities (inferior to the diaphragm).

How do the systems interact?

The 11 organ systems in the human body work together to carry out the functions necessary to life. There are some functions that are true of all complex animals. These include maintaining boundaries, responding to environmental change, moving, ingesting and digesting nutrients, reproducing, growing, removing waste, and utilizing metabolism. Each of these functions as well as some of the organs used for these functions are discussed below.

Maintaining boundaries – The cells in the human body are eukaryotic cells (recall that this means they are surrounded by a membrane as are the organelles inside). Recall that the semi-permeable membrane allows some substances to pass through while restricting others. In addition to this membrane that keeps the internal parts of the cell in the cell and the external parts outside, the integumentary system surrounds the entire body. Recall that the integumentary system serves to protect the internal organs from injury and environmental damage.

Responding to environmental change – The human body has the ability to sense and respond to environmental stimuli involuntarily. For example, think about touching something very hot. You instinctively jerk your hand away. You don't take time to think about what you need to do. From the above discussion, what system is the first responder to these environmental changes? You were correct if you thought of the nervous system. Recall that the nervous system then activates other systems as necessary.

Moving – Recall that the sole purpose of muscular tissue is to move. The muscular system moves the skeletal system to provide voluntary movement. The muscle tissues in the cardiovascular, digestive, reproductive, urinary, and respiratory systems also move. Recall that this movement is involuntary.

Ingestion and digestion – The organs in the digestive system work to remove nutrients from the food we eat and transmit those nutrients to other parts of the body using the cardiovascular system.

Reproduction – While the reproductive system clearly plays a key role in reproduction, hormones must regulate the process. So, the endocrine system works with the reproductive system.

Growing – Growth takes activity from all systems. The skeletal and muscular systems change shape. The digestive system removes nutrients from food. The cardiovascular system moves these nutrients to the cells. The endocrine system must release hormones that signal growth. Give some thought to how the other organ systems play a role in growth.

Excretion – Once the nutrients have been removed in the digestion system, the remains are excreted from the body by organs in both the digestive system (the intestines, rectum and anus) and the urinary system (bladder and urethra).

Metabolism – Recall that metabolism is the way that cells use energy. So, metabolism is the collection of chemical reactions within a cell. The digestive and respiratory systems supply the nutrients and oxygen that the body needs for the metabolism. Of course, the blood distributes these materials throughout the body, and hormones secreted by the glands of the endocrine system regulate the body's metabolism.

When all the needs of the body are being met, the body is in homeostasis. Recall that this means that the body is in a stable state. From the above discussion, you should note that all organ systems are necessary for homeostasis. For example, consider the integumentary system. The skin remains healthy by receiving oxygen and nutrients from the respiratory and digestive systems that travel through blood vessels in the cardiovascular system. The lymphatic system picks up excess fluid from the skin to avoid swelling. The skeletal system provides support. Hormones from the endocrine system regulate hair growth and hydration. The skin serves to protect internal organs, including those in the reproductive system. The muscular system generates heat which is expelled through the skin as sweat, and the urinary system activates vitamin D. The nervous system regulates sweat, interprets stimuli, and adjusts the diameter of blood vessels in the skin.

What are some other ways in which the various organ systems work together? Below are some possibilities. The list is not all inclusive. (Note: The integumentary system was discussed above.)

- **Relationships with the skeletal system**
  - The endocrine system releases hormones that regulate growth and the release of calcium.
  - The lymphatic system contains immune cells that protect against pathogens and removes excess fluid.
  - The digestive system provides nutrients.
  - The urinary system activates vitamin D and removes wastes.
  - The muscular system helps determine bone shape and pulls against the bone to increase bone strength.
  - The nervous system senses pain stimuli in the bones and joints.
  - The respiratory system provides oxygen and removes carbon dioxide.
  - The cardiovascular system supplies oxygen and nutrients while removing waste.
  - The reproductive system influences the skeletal form.
  - The integumentary system provides vitamin D.
- **Relationships with the muscular system**
  - The endocrine system releases hormones that influence strength.
  - The nervous system regulates muscle activity.
  - The reproductive system encourages larger muscle size in men.
  - The bones provide levers for muscular activity.
- **Relationships with the nervous system**
  - The endocrine system releases hormones that regulate the metabolism of neurons.
  - The urinary system helps dispose of metabolic wastes and maintains the correct electrolyte arrangement.
  - Testosterone from the reproductive system stimulates the development of the male reproductive organs, encourages growth of bone and muscle, and helps maintain muscle strength.
- **Relationships with the endocrine system**
  - The cardiovascular system provides a means of transportation for hormones.
  - The muscular system provides protection for some endocrine glands.
  - The nervous system controls the functions of the pituitary gland.
- **Relationships with the cardiovascular system**
  - Hormones released from the endocrine system influence blood pressure.
  - The urinary system helps regulate blood volume and pressure by altering urine volume.
  - The nervous system controls the blood pressure and force, heart rate and blood distribution.
  - In women, estrogen helps preserve vascular health.
  - The integumentary system allows heat to escape.
  - Blood cells are formed in the confines of the skeletal system.
- **Relationships with the lymphatic system**
  - The urinary system helps with proper lymphatic functioning by helping to maintain proper water/ acid-base/ electrolyte balance of the blood.
  - The brain helps control immune response.
  - Acidic secretions in both the reproductive and integumentary systems prevent bacterial growth.
- **Relationships with the respiratory system**
  - The muscular system aids in breathing by producing volume changes (the diaphragm and intercostal muscles).
  - The nervous system regulates breathing rate and depth.
- **Relationships with the digestive system**
  - Increased skeletal muscle activity increases movement of the gastrointestinal tract.
  - The urinary system transforms vitamin D to a form that helps absorption of calcium.

- **Relationships with the urinary system**
  - o   The endocrine system helps regulate re-absorption of water and electrolytes in the renal area.
  - o   The liver (digestive system) synthesizes urea that must be excreted by the kidneys.
- **Relationships with the reproductive system**
  - o   The cardiovascular system transports sex hormones.
  - o   The muscular system is involved in childbirth.
  - o   The respiratory rate increases during pregnancy.

Human Body Science Practice Test

Test Information

The examination you are about to take is multiple choice with only one correct answer per item. Photocopy the answer sheet on this page to record your choices. Circle the correct answers on your answer sheet for each test item. When you have completed the practice test, you may check your answers with those listed on the answer key that follows the Human Body Science Practice Test questions.

Answer Sheet

1.	a	b	c	d			30.	a	b	c	d	e	f
								g	h	i	j	k	
2.	a	b	c	d			31.	a	b	c	d	e	f
3.	a	b	c	d				g	h	i	j	k	
4.	a	b	c	d			32.	a	b	c	d	e	f
5.	a	b	c	d				g	h	i	j	k	
6.	a	b	c	d			33.	a	b	c	d	e	f
7.	a	b	c	d				g	h	i	j	k	
8.	a	b	c	d			34.	a	b	c	d	e	f
9.	a	b	c	d				g	h	i	j	k	
10.	a	b	c	d			35.	a	b	c	d	e	f
11.	a	b	c	d				g	h	i	j	k	
12.	a	b	c	d			36.	a	b	c	d	e	f
13.	a	b	c	d				g	h	i	j	k	
14.	a	b	c	d			37.	a	b	c	d	e	f
15.	a	b	c	d				g	h	i	j	k	
16.	a	b	c	d			38.	a	b	c	d	e	f
17.	a	b	c	d				g	h	i	j	k	
18.	a	b	c	d			39.	a	b	c	d	e	f
19.	a	b	c	d				g	h	i	j	k	
20.	a	b	c	d			40.	a	b	c	d	e	f
21.	a	b	c	d				g	h	i	j	k	
22.	a	b	c	d			41.	a	b	c	d	e	f
23.	a	b	c	d				g	h	i	j	k	
24.	a	b	c	d			42.	a	b	c	d	e	f
25.	a	b	c	d				g	h	i	j	k	
26.	a	b	c	d			43.	a	b	c	d	e	f
27.	a	b	c	d	e	f		g	h	i	j	k	
	g	h	i	j	k		44.	a	b	c	d	e	f
28.	a	b	c	d	e	f		g	h	i	j	k	
	g	h	i	j	k		45.	a	b	c	d	e	f
29.	a	b	c	d	e	f		g	h	i	j	k	
	g	h	i	j	k								

Human Body Science Practice Test

Answer the following items.

1. The knee is _____ to the femur.
   a. distal
   b. lateral
   c. anterior
   d. proximal

2. The heart is _____ to the sternum.
   a. deep
   b. inferior
   c. distal
   d. lateral

3. The pelvic cavity is _____ to the thoracic cavity.
   a. inferior
   b. superficial
   c. medial
   d. anterior

4. The bladder is part of the:
   a. cardiovascular system.
   b. nervous system.
   c. urinary system.
   d. muscular system.

5. The spine is part of the:
   a. skeletal system.
   b. nervous system.
   c. lymphatic system.
   d. endocrine system.

6. Muscular tissue includes all of the following EXCEPT:
   a. skeletal muscle.
   b. nervous muscle.
   c. cardiac muscle.
   d. smooth muscle.

Answer questions 7 and 8 by using the diagram.

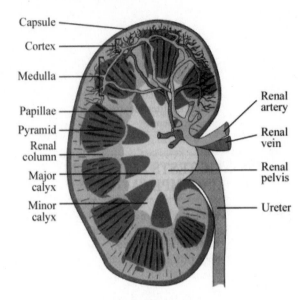

7. The mechanism for urine formation is presented in the figure. Which of the following statements is true?
    a. The renal vein brings nutrients into the kidney.
    b. The kidney is part of the reproductive system.
    c. The kidney helps maintain blood composition.
    d. The ureter takes wastes to the rectum.

8. The diagram shows a(n):
    a. sagittal section.
    b. frontal section.
    c. transverse section.
    d. anterior section.

Questions 9 through 12 refer to the cardiovascular system.

The cardiovascular system is composed of the heart and blood vessels. The heart pumps blood from the left side of the heart into the major arteries. The arteries transport oxygenated blood under pressure to the tissues through the capillaries. The veins carry deoxygenated blood from the tissues back to the right side of the heart, to be circulated through the pulmonary system for oxygenation. Blood volume varies with body weight. Arterial blood pressure is directly related to volume and force. The circulatory process is presented below.

Pump →	Connecting vessels →	Blood →	Tissue contact
(Heart)	(Arteries/veins)	(Cell nutrients) (Osmosis/diffusion)	

Use the figure of the heart to answer questions 9-12.

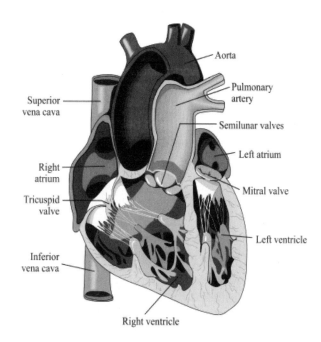

9. If the mitral valve was *prolapsed* (had fallen or slipped from its usual position), which problem should you anticipate?
   a. backup of blood in the left atrium
   b. backup of blood in the right atrium
   c. incomplete emptying of the right ventricle
   d. incomplete emptying of the right atrium

10. The relationship between the inferior vena cava and the aorta is the:
    a. vena cava is connected with the aorta.
    b. vena cava is on the opposite side of the aorta.
    c. aorta is parallel to the vena cava.
    d. aorta is on the back of the heart, vena cava is on the front.

11. Which type of tissue would you find in the heart?
    a. connective
    b. cardiac muscle
    c. simple epithelium
    d. both a and b

12. The pulmonary artery is _____ to the left ventricle.
    a. anterior
    b. inferior
    c. superior
    d. medial

Questions 13 through 15 relate to the neurological system.

The nervous system is frequently described as an electrical conduction system because, through mechanical and chemical stimuli, messages are carried by nerves to all parts of the body for a response. The structure and design of nervous tissue and organs support this concept of communication. All nerve cells have dendrites which receive stimuli from the external and internal environments and bring them to the neurons for interpretation. Another structure, the axon, leaves the neuron to carry the response to the appropriate place. The central nervous system includes the brain and spinal cord. The peripheral nervous system consists of 12 pairs of cranial nerves and 31 pairs of spinal nerves. The autonomic nervous system includes two types of nerves, sympathetic (active when person is excited) and parasympathetic (active when person is at rest), which have opposite effects on the body, thereby maintaining homeostasis. The neurological process for integrating voluntary and involuntary activities is represented below:

Stimulation →	Conduction →	Interpretation →	Response
(Sensory mechanisms)	(Cell nutrients) (Osmosis/diffusion)	(Brain)	(Motor mechanisms)

Structure of a Typical Neuron

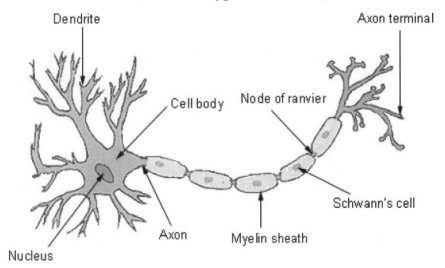

13. Which of the following activities is most likely controlled by the nervous system?
    a. Remove heat from the blood
    b. Regulate blood pressure
    c. Provide nutrients to various parts of the body
    d. Control muscle growth

14. Which is NOT a protection for the brain?
    a. skull
    b. cerebrospinal fluid
    c. blood-brain barrier
    d. smooth muscle

15. Which characteristic is common to both the conduction of nerve impulses and the conduction of an electrical current?
    a. energy output measured by volts
    b. charge affected by positive and negative ions
    c. creates a magnetic field
    d. must be grounded

Questions 16 and 17 refer to the digestive system.

The purpose of the digestive tract (alimentary canal) is to receive and prepare food for metabolism. The breaking down of food includes both a mechanical (e.g., chewing) and a chemical (e.g., enzyme) process. The smooth muscle is stimulated by both parasympathetic and sympathetic nerve fibers. The peristaltic movement helps to mix food with digestive juices. The stomach is able to hold large quantities of food until it can be moved into the small intestines. The pancreas secretes insulin and enzymes into the duodenum, while the liver secretes bile and receives all nutrients through the portal system to contribute to the metabolic process. Wastes are eliminated through the large intestine (colon).

The process of digestion is represented below:

Intake →	Passageway →	Breakdown →	Absorption →	Elimination
(Quantity and quality)	(Patency peristalsis)	(Chemical and mechanical)	(diffusion into blood)	(Water and byproducts of catabolism)

16. Peristalsis propels food through the digestive system by contraction of which muscle type?
    a. skeletal
    b. cardiac
    c. nervous
    d. smooth

17. What substance is absorbed in the small intestine?
    a. oxygen
    b. fats
    c. hormones
    d. lymph tissue

Questions 18-20 relate to these nutritional principles.

Life-maintaining activities of the body cells are dependent on nutrition. Each nutrient has a specific function. The quantity of food supply to the tissues determines the efficiency of the tissue functioning.

18. The most rapid way to reduce caloric intake is to:
    a. reduce fats.
    b. reduce carbohydrates.
    c. increase proteins.
    d. increase water intake.

19. Which of the following statements is a misconception?
    a. Acid-base balance can be regulated by diet.
    b. Blood analysis is the main index for evaluating nutritional status.
    c. Inadequate intake or digestion of one type of nutrient will bring about changes in the remaining nutrients.
    d. If you increase your vitamin intake, you can lessen your basic food intake.

20. A person is described as "wasting away" because of rapid weight loss. Which of the following assumptions can be made?
    a. The person is not eating enough calories.
    b. The person needs supplemental vitamins and minerals.
    c. Proteins are being used as the primary caloric source.
    d. The person's metabolic rate is low.

In the diagram, A is the clavicle, B is the sacrum, C is the patella, D is the femur, E is the scapula, F is the tibia, and G is the radius. Use this information to answer questions 21 and 22.

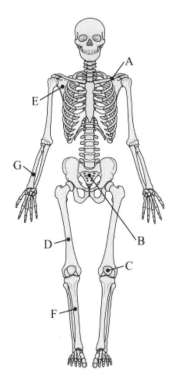

21. If a person has a torn ligament of the radius you would expect:
    a. spasms of the arm.
    b. inability to rotate the wrist.
    c. loss of sensation.
    d. exposure of the elbow cartilage.

22. If the tibia is broken, one would expect restricted movement of the:
    a. patella.
    b. toes.
    c. femur.
    d. ligaments in the leg.

23. The role of vitamin D in the growth and development of bone is best described as:
    a. controlling phosphorus and Ca levels.
    b. regulating the utilization of mineral salts.
    c. promoting Ca absorption.
    d. inhibiting Ca absorption.

24. Which statement is true?
    a. The arrangement of fibers within a muscle determines the capacity of forceful contraction.
    b. Visceral muscle is under voluntary control.
    c. The functional unit of muscle tissue is sarcoplasm.
    d. The more muscle cells innervated, the finer the movement.

Questions 25 and 26 relate to how the organ systems work together.

25. How does the integumentary system work with the digestive system?
     a.   The digestive system provides nutrients for the integumentary system.
     b.   The integumentary system supplies movement for the digestive system.
     c.   The integumentary system removes heat generated by the digestive system.
     d.   The digestive system removes wastes from the integumentary system.

26. The reproductive system works with other organ systems by:
     a.   influencing bone growth and form.
     b.   releasing hormones that influence muscle strength.
     c.   controlling the pituitary gland.
     d.   removing some wastes from the lymphatic system.

In questions 27-45, match the organ system function with the organ system. Some will be used more than once.

     a.   Endocrine system
     b.   Lymphatic system
     c.   Integumentary system
     d.   Skeletal system
     e.   Cardiovascular system
     f.   Reproductive system
     g.   Urinary system
     h.   Digestive system
     i.   Nervous system
     j.   Muscular system
     k.   Respiratory system

27. Removes nitrogen-containing wastes from the body
28. Waterproofs the body
29. Supplies the body with oxygen and removes carbon dioxide
30. Supplies the body cells with oxygen and nutrients and remove wastes
31. Directs bodily defenses against external stimuli
32. Regulates heart and breathing rates
33. Releases hormones that influence strength
34. Regulates electrolyte balance
35. Regulates re-absorption of water and electrolytes
36. Transforms vitamin D into a useful form
37. Serves as mineral storage
38. Releases heat built up by the muscular system
39. Provides motion
40. Provides nutrients for the body and removes wastes
41. Transports hormones throughout the body
42. Controls functions of the pituitary gland
43. Underlies aggressive behavior in the brain
44. Absorbs vitamin D from the external environment
45. Regulates muscle growth

END OF THE TEST

Human Body Science Explanatory Answers

1. a   Recall that distal means further from the trunk of the body.

2. a   The heart is underneath the sternum.

3. a   The pelvic cavity is below the thoracic cavity.

4. c   The bladder is part of the urinary system.

5. a   The spine is the bony protection for the spinal cord.

6. b   Nervous tissue composes the nervous system; it isn't called nervous muscle.

7. c   The kidney helps maintain blood composition by maintaining water, acid-base, and electrolyte balance, and allowing nitrogen-containing wastes to be excreted in urine.

8. b   This is a frontal section.

9. a   The mitral valve is on the left side of the heart separating the ventricle and atrium. If it prolapsed, the blood would back up.

10. b   Recall that inferior means toward the lower part of the body.

11. d   Remember that blood is connective tissue and the heart is cardiac muscle.

12. c   The pulmonary artery is above the left ventricle.

13. b   The nervous system helps regulate heart rate and blood pressure.

14. d   Internal organs are composed of smooth muscle.

15. b   The transmission of nerve impulses (current) is conducted through one exchange of positive and negative ion, inside and outside of the nerve membranes, triggering an electrical signal to the next cell.

16. d   Smooth muscle is found in the digestive system. Contractions of the smooth muscle (peristalsis) force contractions of the digestive system.

17. b   Absorption of fats doesn't begin until the contents reach the small intestine. By the time the contents have passed from one end of the small intestine to the other, almost all food absorption has occurred.

18. a   The energy value is 9 calories per gram for fats and 4 calories per gram for carbohydrates and proteins.

19. d   Vitamins are only effective when combined with balanced nutrients, otherwise they are simply excreted through the digestive track.

20. c   When calories are not available from fat and carbohydrate metabolism, the body will use proteins for the primary source of calories.

21. b   The ligament connecting the radius and the ulna permits rotation of the radius around the ulna.

22. b   One would expect the movement of the bones, muscles, and ligaments distal to the break to be impeded.

23. c   Vitamin D is required for absorption of calcium from the intestine. While Vitamin D also promotes absorption of phosphorus, the reduced phosphorus absorption seen in Vitamin D deficiency is secondary to the reduced absorption of calcium.

24.	a	Visceral (smooth) muscle is under involuntary (autonomic) control. The functional unit of striated muscle tissue is the sarcomere. Precision of movement depends on type of muscle as well as innervation. The force of muscle contraction is dependent on the density of muscle fibers.
25.	a	The digestive system provides nutrients for all organ systems.
26.	a	The reproductive system influences differences in skeletal form seen in men and women.

27. g
28. c
29. k
30. e
31. i
32. i
33. a
34. g
35. a
36. g
37. d
38. c
39. j
40. h
41. e
42. i
43. f
44. c
45. f

Chemical and Physical Science

Some basic chemistry was discussed earlier. We will begin here with a short review of scientific measurement, chemical quantities, and states of matter.

There are two types of measurement that are important in science. There is numerical measurement and descriptive measurement. **Quantitative measurement** is useful when a numerical result is used. This type of measurement allows for measurement comparison at different times. **Qualitative measurements** are less precise because only description or qualities are reported. An example of quantitative measurement of temperature would be "72°F," while a qualitative measurement would be "warm."

Quantitative measurements in science can often be very small numbers or very large numbers. For simplicity, **scientific notation** is used in recording these numbers. In scientific notation, a number is written as a product of a number between 1.00 and 9.99 and 10 raised to some power. Below are some examples of numbers written in the typical form and in scientific notation.

Number	Explanation	Scientific notation
3527	To write this as a number between 1 and 9, there has to be a decimal placed between the 3 and 5. For that to happen, think about what would have to be multiplied by 3.527 to return to 3527. So, if you multiplied by 1000 (or 10^3), the 3.527 would return to 3527.	$3.527 \times 10^3 = 3527$
490,250	This time, there will be a decimal between the 4 and 9. Begin counting to the left from the "invisible decimal" that is right behind the last 0 to find that we will need to multiply by 100,000 (or 10^5) to return to the typical writing.	4.9025×10^5
0.3452	To get this number to something between 1 and 9, we have to move the decimal one place to the right. If you have to move to the right, the exponent will be NEGATIVE!	3.452×10^{-1}
0.000056	Remember that the goal is to represent the number as something between 1.00 and 9.99. Here, that means we want a decimal between the 5 and 6.	$5.6 \times 10^{-5} - 0.000056$

It is often necessary to perform numerical operations on numbers written in scientific notation. While one could translate the numbers back to their typical representations, perform the operations, and then translate back, such a procedure wastes effort. Let's quickly review the rules when working with exponents: Numbers can only be added or subtracted if they have the same exponent. When multiplying two numbers with exponents, add the exponents. When dividing two numbers with exponents, subtract the exponents (bottom from top).

Examples of numerical operations in scientific notation:

1. Multiplication.

$$(3.4 \times 10^2)(1.2 \times 10^7) = (3.4 \times 1.2)(10^2 \times 10^7) = (3.4 \times 1.2)(10^{2+7}) = 4.08 \times 10^9$$

2. Division.

$$\left(\frac{1.7208 \times 10^8}{4.78 \times 10^3}\right) = \left(\frac{17.208 \times 10^7}{4.78 \times 10^3}\right) = \left(\frac{17.208}{4.78}\right)\left(\frac{10^7}{10^3}\right) = \left(\frac{17.208}{4.78}\right)(10^{7-3}) = 3.6 \times 10^4$$

Notice that before dividing, 1.7208 was changed to 17.208 and the exponent was lowered to 7. Another option would be to work the problem as is and then alter the answer so that it is represented by an number between 1 and 9.

$$\left(\frac{1.7208 \times 10^8}{4.78 \times 10^3}\right) = \left(\frac{1.7208}{4.78}\right)\left(\frac{10^8}{10^3}\right) = \left(\frac{1.7208}{4.78}\right)(10^{8-3}) = 0.36 \times 10^5 = 3.6 \times 10^4$$

3. Addition/ Subtraction.

$$(3.5709 \times 10^5) + (5.789 \times 10^4) = (35.709 \times 10^4) + (5.789 \times 10^4) =$$
$$(35.709 + 5.789)(10^4 + 10^4) = 41.498 \times 10^4 = 4.1498 \times 10^5$$

Notice here that the exponents do not change when adding occurs. The final answer, again, must be a number between 1 and 9. For this to occur, the exponent must be increased by one because the decimal moves one place to the left.

Regardless of the measurement, there will always be some uncertainty. Accuracy and precision are two concepts necessary in scientific measurement. **Accuracy** is a reflection of how near the actual measurement the taken measure is. **Precision** is a reflection of how close multiple measurements are to one another. It is possible to have both, one or the other, or neither. The diagrams below show all four options. From left to right: precise but not accurate, neither precise nor accurate, accurate but not precise, both accurate and precise.

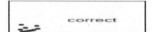 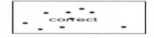 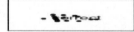 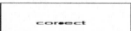

Density is the mass of the object in relation to its volume. If an object's mass is measured in grams and its volume is measured in milliliters, then the object's density is measured in grams per milliliter. Substances that are less dense float in substances that are more dense. Consider ice cubes in a glass of water. The solid water floats because it is less dense than the liquid water. Similarly, a helium balloon floats in the air because helium is less dense than the surrounding air.

Chemical Quantities

In chemistry, a unit called a **mole** is often used to discuss the quantity of a substance. A mole is 6.02×10^{23} representative particles of a substance (that is, atoms, molecules or other units). The concept of counting particles was proposed by Amedeo Avogadro di Quaregna and is called Avogadro's number in his honor. The mass in grams of a substance is the **molar mass** of substance. Calculations in terms of moles are often done in chemistry. However, that is beyond the scope of this review.

Atomic Structure

Matter is anything that takes up space and has mass. Remember, mass is NOT the same as weight. **Mass** is simply the quantity of matter an object has. Substances that cannot be broken into simpler types of matter are called **elements**. All known elements are arranged in a specific order on the periodic table. An **atom** is the smallest part of an element that still retains all the original properties of the element.

The basic structure of an atom is the same for all atoms. All atoms have a **nucleus** (central core) comprised of protons and neutrons. Protons are particles with a positive electrical charge. Neutrons have no electrical charge – they are neutral! The number of protons is the same for any atom of the same element. The **atomic number** of an element is the number of protons in the nucleus of an atom of the element. The atomic number serves as an ordering device for the periodic table. The third type of particle within an atom is called an **electron**. An electron has a negative charge. In most atoms, there are an equal number of protons and electrons so that the overall charge is zero. Electrons do not reside in the nucleus of an atom. Instead, electrons orbit the nucleus in **energy levels**. Each energy level can hold a limited number of electrons. The number of levels depends on the element. Usually, an atom is not stable by itself. Atoms are only stable when their outermost energy level is full. So, the atoms of one element tend to easily combine with atoms of another element. When atoms of one element are combined with atoms of another element, the result is a **molecule** of a compound.

Elements combine with other elements to form **compounds**. Compounds do not necessarily have the same physical properties of the individual elements. Consider water. Water is really a combination of the two gaseous elements oxygen and hydrogen. Once the two elements combine into the compound water, the compound is a liquid.

To combine, atoms undergo **chemical reactions** to come to a stable state. In the reactions, some chemical bonds are broken, the atoms rearrange, and new attachments (**bonds**) are formed. There are two kinds of chemical bonds. If two or more atoms share one or more pairs of electrons, the bond is called covalent. The other kind of bond, an ionic bond, occurs when an electron from one atom is transferred to an atom of another element. This transfer results in atoms with electrical charges (one positive and one negative). An atom with an electrical charge is an **ion**. This attraction between the positive and negative ion is the **ionic bond**.

There are several types of chemical reactions that occur in any organism. A chemical reaction that yields a net release of **free energy** (energy that can be used for work within a system) is a **exergonic reaction**. If the reaction yields a net absorption of free energy, it is a **endergonic reaction**. There is a certain amount of energy necessary to begin any chemical reaction. This energy is called activation energy. The amount of activation energy necessary can be decreased if the correct **catalyst** is present. A catalyst is simply a chemical substance that decreases the amount of activation necessary for a chemical reaction. In living things, **enzymes** are a very important group of catalysts. The chemical reactions that result in transference of electrons are **reduction-oxidation reactions** (redox reactions). An **oxidation reaction** occurs when an atom loses one or more electrons, resulting in a positive charge. In a **reduction reaction**, an atom gains one or more electrons, resulting in a negative charge.

Think it Through

1. Describe the construction of an atom.
2. Why does hydrogen gas exists as H_2 and never just as H? (That is, why do two hydrogen atoms need to be connected together in the natural state?)

Answers

1. Atoms contain a nucleus in which protons and neutrons reside. Electrons circle the nucleus in varying energy levels.
2. Hydrogen exists only in pairs because the atom is unstable on its own. A covalent bond is necessary to make the atom stable.

The States of Matter

There are three states of matter: gases, liquids, and solids. Before we discuss them, recall that **kinetic energy** is the energy of an object in motion. The kinetic theory states that particles in all forms of matter are constantly in motion.

The assumptions of the kinetic theory for gasses are that the volume occupied by a gas is mostly empty space. It also assumes that the particles of gas are far apart, move rapidly, and have random motion. **Gas pressure** is just the result of billions of particles colliding with an object simultaneously. If there is an empty space with no particles and no pressure, then there is a **vacuum**.

A **liquid** forms when the temperature of the gas lowers enough for condensation to occur. A liquid can be changed into a gas through **vaporization**. If this process does not include boiling, then **evaporation** is occurring.

A **solid** forms when the temperature lowers even further. The particles in a solid have only very restricted movement about fixed points. The structure of a solid is typically crystalline. This means that the particles that make up the structure are in an orderly, repeating, three-dimensional pattern known as a **crystal lattice**. Some solids exist in different crystalline forms. Think about carbon. It can exist as both a diamond and as graphite. These two forms have different crystalline structures.

Substances typically change from solid to liquid (through melting) and then to gas (through vaporization). However, there are instances when a solid changes directly to a gas without going through a liquid stage. This process is known as sublimation and occurs typically at higher than usual pressure.

Test Information

The examination you are about to take is multiple choice with only one correct answer per item. Photocopy the answer sheet on this page to record your choices. Circle the correct answers on your answer sheet for each test item. When you have completed the practice test, you may check your answers with those listed on the answer key that follows the Chemical and Physical Science Practice Test questions.

Chemical and Physical Science Practice Test
Answer Sheet

1.	a	b	c	d		18.	a	b	c	d
2.	a	b	c	d		19.	a	b	c	d
3.	a	b	c	d		20.	a	b	c	d
4.	a	b	c	d		21.	a	b	c	d
5.	a	b	c	d		22.	a	b	c	d
6.	a	b	c	d		23.	a	b	c	d
7.	a	b	c	d		24.	a	b	c	d
8.	a	b	c	d		25.	a	b	c	d
9.	a	b	c	d		26.	a	b	c	d
10.	a	b	c	d		27.	a	b	c	d
11.	a	b	c	d		28.	a	b	c	d
12.	a	b	c	d		29.	a	b	c	d
13.	a	b	c	d		30.	a	b	c	d
14.	a	b	c	d		31.	a	b	c	d
15.	a	b	c	d		32.	a	b	c	d
16.	a	b	c	d		33.	a	b	c	d
17.	a	b	c	d		34.	a	b	c	d

Chemical and Physical Science Practice Test

Questions 1 and 2 relate to density.

The density of a substance is equal to the mass (amount of matter) of the substance divided by the volume of the substance. Density is an intrinsic property that does not change with the amount of material. Three different liquids with different densities were placed together in a container as shown. The liquids, when stirred and allowed to resettle, returned to the same arrangement.

1. Which statement is true about these liquids?
    a. Liquid 1 has a lower density than Liquid 2.
    b. Liquid 1 has a higher density than Liquid 2.
    c. All three densities may be equal.
    d. No conclusion can be drawn about the relative densities on the basis of the observations.

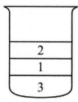

Archimedes' principle states that an object placed under water displaces a volume of water equal to its own volume.

2. If a boy has a pile of small rocks of the same composition and he wants to determine the density (mass/volume) of the rocks, which combination of devices should he use?
    a. A yardstick and a small pan large enough to hold the rocks
    b. A larger pan and a balance
    c. A supply of water and a large measuring graduated cylinder
    d. A balance, a supply of water and a large graduated (measuring) cylinder

Questions 3 and 4 relate to the chemical activity of gases

Gases consist of molecules of specific substances. For instance, a molecule of oxygen is made up of two atoms of oxygen bound together. The relative rates at which the molecules of the two gases move is inversely proportional to the square roots of the densities of the two gases. That is, $\dfrac{\text{Rate of Gas A}}{\text{Rate of Gas B}} = \dfrac{\sqrt{\text{Density}_A}}{\sqrt{\text{Density}_B}}$.

3. If two gases (A and B), which have detectable odors, are released simultaneously on one side of a room and the odor of Gas A is noticed one minute before that of Gas B, which of these conclusions can be a likely explanation?
    a. The odor of A is stronger than that of B.
    b. Gas A has a higher density than that of Gas B.
    c. Gas B has a higher density than Gas A.
    d. The opening in the container of Gas A is larger than that of Gas B.

4. A certain amount of a substance is in a solid state, but is melted to form a liquid and finally vaporized to form a gas. The solid has a volume of one cubic centimeter, the liquid occupies 0.75 cubic centimeters and the gas expands to 10 cubic meters. Which statement is NOT true?
    a. The liquid is more dense than the gas.
    b. The liquid is less dense than the solid.
    c. The solid is more dense than the gas.
    d. The liquid has the highest density of the three forms.

Questions 5 and 6 relate to solutions and concentrations.

The general concept of a solution includes solvents (the host substance) and solutes (the dispersed substance). The abundance of a solution's solute determines its concentration (dilute-concentrated). The amount of solute in a solution can be measured by moles (gram formula weights) and therefore can be described as having a certain molarity. The limit to the concentration of a solution is called its solubility. Different compounds range from insoluble to highly soluble.

5. Prazosin, a neurological medication, was prepared in varying concentrations. A patient was given twice a day treatment of 10^{-4}M dosage. The treatment was ineffective, so the doctor decided to DOUBLE the dosage. This molar concentration is expressed as:
   a. 2×10^{-4}.
   b. 10^{-8}.
   c. 10^{-5}.
   d. 10^{-2}.

6. A scientist is asked to prepare a solution of Trizma-HCl with a concentration of 0.1576 g/L. If a smaller quantity is desired, a technician can conserve chemicals and maintain the same concentration by mixing:
   a. 0.1576 mg/ ml.
   b. 0.1576 mg/10 ml.
   c. 0.1576 g/10 L.
   d. 0.1576 mg/L.

Questions 7 through 11 relate to force, volume, and temperature for a gas

There are specific relationships among force, volume, and temperature. **Charles' Law** states that the volume of a gas varies directly with the absolute temperature, providing the pressure is constant. **Boyle's Law** states that the volume varies inversely with the pressure at a constant temperature.

7. Suppose you had a steel cylinder containing a piston which is resting on a block of ice as shown. The piston could be raised or lowered without allowing any of the air in the cylinder below the piston to escape. To test the hypothesis that the greater the force on the piston (hence the smaller the volume of air), the greater the amount of heat generated, which of the methods below would be most useful?

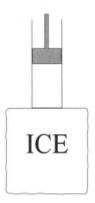

   a. Measure the amount of water produced immediately when the piston is forced down to one-half its original height.
   b. Measure the amount of water produced when the piston is raised to twice its original height.
   c. Measure the amount of water produced within five minutes after the piston has been lowered to each of three different levels in succession.
   d. Choose three lower levels, move the piston from its original position to each position and measure the amount of water produced in each case.

8. If an operating refrigerator is placed in a small insulated room for one hour with its door left open, the room temperature will:
   a. approach freezing during the hour.
   b. remain nearly constant.
   c. increase.
   d. become cooler, but will not approach freezing.

9. The specific heat of a substance is a measure of the quantity of heat required to raise the temperature of one gram of the substance one degree Celsius. Consider that the specific heat (calories/(gram x°C)) of water is 1.0 and 0.215 for aluminum. If an aluminum pan filled with cold water is placed on a burner at 450°F, the:
   a. water heats faster and aluminum cools faster.
   b. water heats faster and aluminum cools slower.
   c. water heats slower and aluminum cools faster.
   d. water and aluminum heat and cool at the same rate.

10. The simple experiment described in question 9 supports the hypothesis that:
    a. water is a better convector of heat than aluminum.
    b. water is a better conductor of heat than aluminum.
    c. aluminum and water conduct heat equally.
    d. the experiment does not address the hypothesis.

A cylinder with an airtight piston was heated in a laboratory where the internal temperature and volume were recorded as follows:

Temperature (K)	Volume
2.0×10^2	20
4.0×10^2	40
6.0×10^2	60
8.0×10^2	80

11. The hypothesis that volume increases proportionally with temperatures at constant pressure was:
    a. refuted by the data.
    b. not related to the data.
    c. obscured by the data.
    d. supported by the data.

Questions 12 through 16 relate to the periodic table.

The periodic table is an arrangement of all known chemical elements in order of their atomic numbers. In each row, the atomic numbers increase toward the right.

I	II	IIIb	IVb	Vb	VIb	VIIb		VIIIb		Ib	IIb	III	IV	V	VI	VII	0
1	2	3	4	5	6	7	8	9	10	11	12	13	14	15	16	17	18
H																	He
Li	Be											B	C	N	O	F	Ne
Na	Mg											Al	Si	P	S	Cl	Ar
K	Ca	Sc	Ti	V	Cr	Mn	Fe	Co	Ni	Cu	Zn	Ga	Ge	As	Se	Br	Kr
Rb	Sr	Y	Zr	Nb	Mo	Tc	Ru	Rh	Pd	Ag	Cd	In	Sn	Sb	Te	I	Xe
Cs	Ba	La*	Hf	Ta	W	Re	Os	Ir	Pt	Au	Hg	Tl	Pb	Bi	Po	At	Rn
Fr	Ra	Ac**	Rf	Db	Sg	Bh	Hs	Mt	Uun	Uuu	Uub		Uuq		Uuh		Uuo

*Lanthanides	Ce	Pr	Nd	Pm	Sm	Eu	Gd	Tb	Dy	Ho	Er	Tm	Yb	Lu
**Actinides	Th	Pa	U	Np	Pu	Am	Cm	Bk	Cf	Es	Fm	Md	No	Lr

12. Of the following four elements, the best electrical conductor is:
   a. Br.
   b. As.
   c. C.
   d. K.

13. Which pair of elements are most alike in reactivity?
   a. Li and K
   b. H and He
   c. Cu and O
   d. Li and He

> Chemical elements can be identified by the number of protons in the nuclei of their atoms (atomic number). The atomic mass is approximately the sum of the neutrons and protons of an atom.

14. All atoms have a neutral charge because negative electrons outside the nuclei balance the positive protons inside the nuclei. Neutrons have no charge. Most elements have isotopes which differ in their atomic masses. The most likely reason for the differences is that the isotopes have different numbers of :
   a. electrons.
   b. protons.
   c. neutrons and protons.
   d. neutrons.

15. The number of neutrons in an isotope with an atomic number of 50 is:
   a. likely to be 50.
   b. likely to exceed 60.
   c. likely to be less than 40.
   d. unpredictable in terms of a comparison with the atomic number.

16. One group of chemical elements referred to as a family has gram atomic weights of approximately 19, 35.5, 79.9, and 126.9. If one of these elements is a solid at room temperature, its gram atomic weight must be:
   a. 19.
   b. 35.5.
   c. 79.9.
   d. 126.9.

Questions 17 and 18 relate to electrochemistry.

Every electric circuit consists of a source for energy, a closed path for the flow of the current, and a device (such as a light bulb) that uses the electrical energy. The number of electrons that flow in the current is called the **amperes**. The pressure produced by the energy source in a circuit is called the **voltage**. The electrons must overcome **electrical resistance** to move through the circuit. A good conductor, such as copper, has low resistance; a poor conductor has high resistance to the flow.

17. When comparing two of the same type of toasters, the one capable of generating the most heat is the one with:
    a.   higher resistance.
    b.   higher current.
    c.   higher voltage and lower resistance.
    d.   higher voltage and higher resistance.

18. An electric current can be carried by movement of electrons and:
    a.   ions.
    b.   atoms.
    c.   photons.
    d.   neutrons.

The strengths of acids and bases are measured on the pH scale, which ranges from 0 to 14. Substances with pH < 7.0 are acids and those > 7.0 are bases.

$$pH = -\log [H^+]$$

Questions 19-22 relate to acid/base balance.

Since the pH scale is expressed as negative logarithms of the H^+ concentration, the smaller the exponent, the greater the acidity. Remember that the logarithm (Base$_{10}$) of a number is the exponential power to which the base must be raised to equal the number in question. Note the following relationship between the $[H^+]$ and $[OH^-]$ concentrations and pH values.

Table: pH Scale		
[H+]	**[pH]**	**[OH-]**
10^{-1}	1.0	10^{-13}
10^{-2}	2.0	10^{-12}
10^{-3}	3.0	10^{-11}
10^{-4}	4.0	10^{-10}
10^{-5}	5.0	10^{-9}
10^{-6}	6.0	10^{-8}
10^{-7}	7.0	10^{-7}
10^{-8}	8.0	10^{-6}
10^{-9}	9.0	10^{-5}
10^{-10}	10.0	10^{-4}
10^{-11}	11.0	10^{-3}
10^{-12}	12.0	10^{-2}
10^{-13}	13.0	10^{-1}
10^{-14}	14.0	10^{-0}

19. A difference of one pH unit represents a concentration difference of:
    a. 1.
    b. 10.
    c. 100.
    d. 1,000.

20. A difference of two pH units represents a concentration difference of:
    a. 2.
    b. 20.
    c. 100.
    d. 1,000.

21. A substance with a pH of 7 when dissolved in water is:
    a. a strong acid.
    b. a weak base.
    c. a neutral salt.
    d. a weak acid.

22. Which of the following characteristics is NOT a property of acids?
    a. sour taste
    b. dissolves metals
    c. turns blue litmus red
    d. liberates OH^- in solution

Questions 23 through 29 relate to force and motion.

It is an established principle of elementary physics that momentum is the product of the mass and the velocity of an object:

$$Momentum = mV \text{ (Velocity = meters/second)}$$

23. An astronaut who lands on the moon will:
    a. have the same mass on the moon as on earth.
    b. have more mass on the moon than on earth.
    c. have less mass on the moon than on earth.
    d. not have measurable mass on the moon.

24. An 8.0 kg car travels at 2.0 m/s. If the driver of a 4.0 kg car traveling at 2.0 m/s wants to generate the same momentum, she could:
    a. add a 4.0 kg object to the vehicle.
    b. increase her velocity to 4.0 m/s.
    c. both a and b.
    d. either a or b.

25. If a metal block is to be raised 10 feet either by hoisting it up directly or by pushing it up a frictionless inclined plane 20 feet long, then:
    a. more work would be done by the direct hoist method.
    b. more work would be done by the inclined plane-push method.
    c. the amount of work by either method is the same.
    d. the amount of force applied to the block is the same in each case.

26. When an automobile traveling at 60 miles per hour is brought to a rapid stop, the two types of energy most involved are:
    a. potential and heat.
    b. potential and kinetic.
    c. kinetic and chemical.
    d. kinetic and heat.

27. If a person swings a ball in a circle and the string breaks near the point of attachment:
    a. the ball will continue moving in the same circle.
    b. the ball will travel in a straight line.
    c. the ball will travel in a wider circle.
    d. the ball will travel in a manner not described above.

28. The motion of the released ball occurs due to:
    a. an absence of centripetal force.
    b. centripetal force.
    c. gravitational acceleration.
    d. kinetic force.

29. If four different people with identical body weights are compared, the person who exerts the least amount of energy is the one who:
    a. runs at a speed of 2 miles per hour.
    b. walks 2 miles slowly.
    c. sits calmly for one hour.
    d. plays touch football for one hour.

Questions 30 through 34 relate to states of matter.

The phase diagram below shows the state(s) a substance is in, depending on conditions of temperature and pressure.

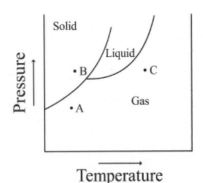

30. Assume that the substance starts in conditions represented by point A. Pressure is then applied until it reaches the state represented by point B. Subsequently the temperature is increased to put the substance in the final state. Which of the following statements is true?
    a. At first, this substance is a liquid.
    b. To go from state B to C, the substance followed the sequence: solid → gas → liquid.
    c. To go from state B to C, the substance followed the sequence: solid → liquid → gas.
    d. Under the final conditions given, the substance was a liquid.

31. Of the following processes, which involve both chemical and physical changes?
    a.   Water is heated to produce steam.
    b.   Papers are cut up in a shredder.
    c.   Hydrogen and oxygen gases react to produce water vapor.
    d.   An egg is hard-boiled.

The boiling point of a liquid is the temperature at which the vapor pressure of the liquid is equal to the atmospheric pressure.

Substances	Boiling Point (°C) at 760 mmHg
Water H_2O	100
Ethanol CH_3CH_2OH	78
Methanol CH_3OH	65
Propanol CH_3CH_2OH	97

32. If the substances in the preceding chart were mixed and fractionally distilled, the order (first-to-last) of recovery would be:
    a.   water, ethanol, methanol, propanol.
    b.   methanol, ethanol, propanol, water.
    c.   ethanol, water, propanol, methanol.
    d.   water, propanol, ethanol, methanol.

33. A student has two material samples. One is supposed to be a metal (A), and the other is supposed to be a non-metal (B). The student is to determine which one is the metal. During the course of observations, which of the following is UNLIKELY to be seen?
    a.   Sample B heated very slowly when heat was applied, but Sample A heated very quickly.
    b.   Sample A cooled rapidly when refrigerated, but Sample B did not.
    c.   Samples A and B both sank when placed in water.
    d.   Samples A and B both conducted an electric current.

34. A student heated 200 ml of water in a 1L tin can. After the water boiled, the student closed the can and allowed it to cool. The student then observed that it crushed from all sides. The demonstration illustrated that:
    a.   air is matter.
    b.   a vacuum was created outside the can.
    c.   the can was weak.
    d.   greater pressure was on the outside of the can.

END OF THE TEST

Chemical and Physical Science Answers and Explanations

1. b   Liquid 1 has a higher density than Liquid 2. A liquid with less density than that of another liquid will float on the latter liquid if these two are placed together. Liquid 3 is therefore the most dense of the three liquids shown.

2. d   Mass (by weighing) and volume (by water displacement) must both be determined in order to obtain the density of the rocks. Therefore, the scale, water, and a graduated cylinder large enough to hold the rocks are all necessary for the density determination.

3. c   Since B has a higher density than A, it would travel more slowly. Consequently molecules of A would reach the other side of the room sooner than molecules of B.

4. b $Density = \dfrac{Mass}{Volume}$ Since the mass is constant in this example, the phase with the smallest volume has the greatest density. The liquid has the highest density

5. a   The original dosage was expressed in exponential terms, but a simple doubling requires multiplication by two.

6. a   The concentration of 0.1576 g/L is the equivalent to 0.1576 mg/ml because 1.0 mg is 10^{-3}g, and 1 ml is 10^{-3}L.

7. d   An increase in pressure with a decrease in volume should cause a temperature increase in each case. The method used in D would give the best chance to show this.

8. c   Energy is required for refrigeration. The gas used for compression during refrigeration releases heat when it is compressed. This heat produced is greater than the cooling power of the open refrigerator. The cooling power is not 100% efficient.

9. c   The unequal heating of water and aluminum is because water is a poor conductor of heat, which enables it to act as a heat regulator in living systems.

10. d   No provision was made to distinguish between heat conduction and heat convection.

11. d   There was a proportional rise in volume as the temperature was increased.

12. d   Metals are good conductors, but nonmetals are not. Potassium (K) is the only metal in the group.

13. a   Elements in columns (or families) on the periodic table have similar electronic structure and, therefore, similar chemistry.

14. d   The number of protons (and electrons) is responsible for the chemical behavior of atoms. Neutrons just add mass and therefore are responsible for differences in isotopes of a given element.

15. b   As elements increase in atomic numbers, the neutron-to-proton ratio tends to increase.

16. d   Elements in a periodic table group tend to progress from gas to liquid to solid (if all three states exist) as atomic numbers increase.

17. d   The combination of high voltage and high resistance will lead to the highest heat production.

18. a   Both negatively and positively charged ions (as well as electrons) can carry electric current; however, neutrally charged atoms, protons, and neutrons do not.

19. b   A difference of one pH unit represents a difference of 10 in strength of concentration in acid because the scale uses $\log_{10}$ units.

20. c   A difference of two pH units represents a difference of 100 in strength of concentration, based on $\log_{10}$.

21. c   A substance with a pH of 7.0 is a neutral salt $[H^+] = 10^{-7}$, $[OH^-] = 10^{-7}$.

22. d   The liberation of OH^- ions in aqueous solutions is a property of bases.

23. a   The mass of an object is a constant, independent of the pull of gravity on that object.

24. d   Increase momentum by doubling velocity = 4 m/s x 4.0 kg = 16 kg·m/s. Alternatively, with the addition of 4 kg, it becomes 8 kg x 2 m/s = 16 kg·m/s.

25. c   The total energy of the block after being lifted is the same if the height to which it has been lifted is the same. However, less force must be applied against the block as it is pushed along the inclined plane than is needed for a direct vertical lift.

26. d   The automobile has energy of motion (kinetic energy) until it stops. In order to stop it relies on friction. The friction generates heat during the course of braking.

27. b   While the ball is being swung it is held in a circle by centripetal force. Without centripetal force (because the string has broken), the ball follows a straight line.

28. a   As mentioned above, without centripetal force, the ball must follow a straight line.

29. c   Any extra physical activity such as walking or running requires more energy than basal metabolism.

30. c   According to the graph, a horizontal movement from point B to point C would carry the substance from solid to liquid to gas.

31. d   The chemical change involves the denaturing of the proteins. The physical change is from a liquid to a solid state.

32. b   Water is recovered last because it has the highest boiling point. The other three substances are alcohols and their boiling points increase with increasing molecular weight.

33. d   In contrast to non-metals, metals absorb and release heat quickly. Metals also are excellent conductors of electricity whereas non-metals are not. Many solids, both metals and non-metals, are dense enough to sink in water.

34. a   This experiment demonstrated that the air which initially filled the can was matter in the gaseous state. Heating the can forced the air molecules out and created a partial vacuum inside when the water vapor condensed back to liquid. The inside pressure was less than the external pressure on the can. The outside air flowed down its pressure gradient and crushed the can.

General Science

Just as the systems within the body work together and follow specific patterns of change, the earth follows certain predictable patterns and cycles. In particular, the hydrologic cycle, the rock cycle, and the theory of plate tectonics are important to our understanding of the earth.

The Hydrologic Cycle

The hydrologic cycle is the process whereby water continually circulates between the earth's surface and atmosphere. Heat energy from the sun provides energy for the cycle. Water from the earth's oceans, lakes, and rivers is warmed by the sun and **evaporates**, returning to the atmosphere as water vapor. As water vapor rises, it cools and **condenses** from vapor back into water droplets. These suspended water droplets may form clouds or fog. Eventually, the temperature and atmospheric pressure cause **precipitation**, the return of water to the earth's surface in the form of rain, sleet, snow, or ice. Precipitation may eventually return to the ocean through streams and rivers as **surface runoff**; or, it may soak into, or **infiltrate**, the soil. Eventually water that returns to the ocean will evaporate again as the water cycle repeats. Another way that water vapor returns to the atmosphere is through **transpiration**; plants absorb water from the soil and return it to the atmosphere through this process.

The Rock Cycle

The rock cycle is a group of changes that transform one type of rock into another. The three rock types are:
1.   Igneous – made when **magma**, a hot liquid made of melted minerals, cools. Magma can cool slowly underground, or quickly on the earth's surface, where it is called lava.
2.   Sedimentary – formed when sediments, pieces of rocks broken off by weathering and erosion, are compacted and cemented together
3.   Metamorphic – formed when rock is transformed by heat and pressure.

Rocks are broken down to become sediment through **weathering.** There are two types of weathering processes. **Physical weathering** causes the disintegration of rocks and minerals through some physical or mechanical process, while **chemical weathering** causes the rocks and minerals to undergo a chemical change or decomposition. Some examples of physical weathering include plant and animal activities, exposure to heat such as a fire, or wedging, when freezing water in the cracks of a rock expands and exerts force on the rock. When rocks that were originally formed beneath the earth's surface are exposed to conditions on the surface, chemical weathering may occur. Water and acids in water are the main agents of chemical weathering.

The heat and pressure necessary to create metamorphic rock is one result of **tectonic plate movement**. The theory of tectonic plate movement states that the outer layer of earth's surface is broken into seven large plates and several smaller ones. The plates move in different directions at different speeds. The plates meet at **plate boundaries.** Boundaries are described in terms of the plates' motion relative to each other. A **convergent boundary** is where two plates are moving against, or toward, each other. A **divergent boundary** is where to plates pull apart. A **transform boundary** is one where two plates are sliding past each other. Some very interesting natural phenomena, including mountain formation, volcanoes, and earthquakes, occur at plate boundaries.

Science Glossary

Acetylcholine (ACH)— chemical transmitter substance released by some nerve endings

Acid— a compound that yields H^+ ions in solution or a solution with the concentration of H^+ exceeding OH^-

Acid-base balance— situation in which the pH of the blood is maintained between 7.35 and 7.45

Actinides— the row of elements below the periodic table, from thorium to lawrencium

Action potential— a large transient depolarization event, including polarity reversal, that is conducted along the membrane of a muscle cell or a nerve fiber

Active transport— membrane transport processes for which ATP is provided (e.g., solute pumping and endocytosis)

Adaptation— receive, interpret, and respond to internal and external stimuli via the nervous system

Adhesion— molecular attraction between dissimilar molecules; attraction between water molecules and molecules that make up the inside of a xylem tube

Adrenergic fibers— nerve fibers that release norepinephrine

Aerobic— in the presence of oxygen

Afferent (sensory) nerve— nerve that contains processes of sensory neurons and carries nerve impulses to the central nervous system

Agglutination— clumping of (foreign) cells; induced by crosslinking of antigen-antibody complexes

Agonist— muscle that bears the major responsibility for effecting a particular movement; a prime mover

Alkali metals— the column of elements from lithium to francium

Allele—any of the alternative forms of a gene

Allergy (hypersensitivity)— overzealous immune response to an otherwise harmless antigen

Alpha particle— a cluster of 2 protons and 2 neutrons emitted from a nucleus in one type of radioactivity

Amnion— fetal membrane that forms a fluid-filled sac around the embryo

Anabolism— energy-requiring building phase of metabolism in which simpler substances are combined to form more complex substances

Anaerobic— without the presence of oxygen

Androgen— a hormone that controls male secondary sex characteristics, such as testosterone

Anion— an atom or molecule with a negative charge

Anode— the negative electrode at which oxidation occurs

Antibody— a protein molecule that is released by a plasma cell (a daughter cell of an activated B lymphocyte) and that binds specifically to an antigen; an immunoglobulin

Aqueous— refers to a solution with water as the solvent

Arteries— blood vessels that conduct blood away from the heart and into circulation

Articulation (joint)— the junction of two or more bones

Asexual reproduction— method of reproducing a new organism from only one parent by means of mitosis

Atom— the smallest amount of an element; a nucleus containing protons and neutrons surrounded by electrons

Atomic number— the number of protons in the nucleus of the chemical element

Atomic weight—the weight in grams of one mole of the chemical element; approximately the number of protons and neutrons in the nucleus

Atrophy— reduction in size or wasting away of an organ or cell resulting from disease or lack of use

Avogadro's Law— equal volumes of gases contain the same number of molecules

Axon— neuron process that carries impulses away from the nerve cell body; efferent process; the conducting portion of a nerve cell

Bactericidal— able to kill bacteria

Basal metabolic rate (BMR)— rate at which energy is expended (heat produced) by the body per unit of time under controlled (basal) conditions: 12 hours after a meal, at rest

Base— a compound that yields OH^- ions in solution or a solution with the concentration of OH^- exceeding H^+

Beta particle— an electron emitted from a nucleus in one type of radioactivity

Blood pressure— force exerted by blood against a unit area of the blood vessel walls; differences in blood pressure between different areas of the circulation provide the driving force for blood circulation

Boiling point— the temperature at which a liquid changes to a gas

Bowman's capsule— a network of capillaries encased in a membrane in the kidney for purpose of filtration

Boyle's Law— the volume of a gas varies inversely with pressure

Bronchioles— the branching air passageways inside the lungs

Buffer— chemical substance or system that minimizes changes in pH by releasing or binding hydrogen ions

Calorie— a unit of energy, equal to 4.184 joules; the energy required to increase the temperature of 1.0 g of water by one degree Celsius

Capillary action— the rising of a liquid in a small tube because of adhesive and cohesive forces

Carbohydrate— organic compound containing carbon, hydrogen, and oxygen. The hydrogen-to-oxygen ratio is 2:1

Catalyst— a chemical that changes the rate of a chemical reaction without itself being chemically altered

Cathode— the positive electrode at which reduction occurs

Cation— an atom or molecule with a positive charge

Charles' Law— the volume of a gas varies directly with temperature

Chlorophyll— green plant pigment that is found in chloroplast and is necessary for photosynthesis

Chloroplast— plant cell structures containing light-sensitive chlorophyll

Circulation— transporting oxygen and other nutrients to the tissues via cardiovascular system

Clone— descendants of a single cell

Coenzyme— nonprotein substance associated with and activating an enzyme, typically a vitamin

Cohesion— attraction between similar molecules (e.g., attraction between two water molecules)

Colloid— suspension that does not separate on standing

Colloidal osmotic pressure— pressure created in a fluid by large non-diffusible molecules, such as plasma proteins, that are prevented from moving through a (capillary) membrane; such substances tend to draw water to them

Colony— group of bacteria cells

Complemental air— amount of air that can be forcefully inhaled

Compound— a substance formed by the chemical combination of two or more elements

Concentration— the relative abundance of a solute in a solution

Corticosteroids— steroid hormones released by the adrenal cortex

Cotyledon— seed leaf that stores food for a plant embryo of seed plants

Covalent bond— atoms linked together by sharing valence electrons

Cranial nerves— the 12 nerve pairs that arise from the brain

Culture medium— specially prepared nutritious substance used to grow experimental organisms

Cytoplasm— the cellular material surrounding the nucleus and enclosed by the plasma membrane

Decomposition— a chemical reaction in which a compound is broken down into simpler compounds or elements

Dehydrate— to lose water

Dendrite— branching neurons that transmit the nerve impulse toward the cell body

Disaccharide— sugar formed by the combination of two simple sugar molecules

DNA (deoxyribonucleic acid)— a nucleic acid found in all living cells which carries the organism's hereditary information

DNA replication— the process that occurs before cell division and insures that all daughter cells have identical genes

Dominant traits— occur when one allele masks or suppresses the expression of its partner

Ecosystem— the interaction of living organisms with their environment

Electrode— a conducting substance that connects an electrolyte to an external circuit

Electrolyte— an ionic substance that has high electrical conductivity

Electron— a light subatomic particle with negative charge; found in orbitals surrounding an atomic nucleus

Element— a substance that cannot be decomposed by ordinary chemical means; each chemical element is characterized by the number of protons in the nucleus (for example, all atoms of hydrogen have 1 proton, and atoms of oxygen have 8 protons)

Elimination— removing metabolic wastes from the body via renal system

Embryo— early development of an animal or a plant after fertilization; cylindrical structure within a seed that develops into a plant

Emulsion— suspension of two liquids which are incapable of mixing or attaining homogeneity

Endocrine glands— ductless glands that empty their hormonal products directly into the blood

Endocrine system— body system that includes internal organs that secrete hormones

Energy— the concept of motion or heat

Enzyme— protein catalyst; chemical that changes the rate of a chemical reaction in living tissue without itself being chemically altered

Equilibrium— a balanced condition resulting from two opposing reactions

Erythrocytes— red blood cells

Estrogen— hormones that stimulate female secondary sex characteristics; female sex hormones

Expiration — process of breathing out

Extracellular fluid— internal fluid located outside cells

Faraday's Laws— two laws of electrolysis relating the amount of substance to the quantity of electric charge

Fascia — layers of fibrous tissue covering and separating muscle

Fermentation— release of energy from sugar without the use of oxygen; anaerobic respiration

Fertilization— fusion of the sperm and egg nuclei

Fetus— developmental stage extending from the ninth week of development to birth

Fibrinogen— a blood protein that is converted to fibrin (a white, insoluble protein) during blood clotting

Filtrate— liquid that passes through the pores in a filter

Follicle— ovarian structure consisting of a developing egg surrounded by one or more layers of follicle cells; colloid-containing structure of the thyroid gland

Follicle stimulating hormone (FSH) — hormone produced by the anterior pituitary that stimulates ovarian follicle production in females and sperm production in males

Free energy— the thermodynamic quantity measuring the tendency of a reaction to proceed; also called Gibbs free energy

Freezing point— the temperature at which a liquid changes to a solid

Fulcrum— the fixed point on which a lever moves when a force is applied

Gamete— sex or germ cell

Genetic code— the rules by which the base sequence of a DNA gene is translated into protein structures (amino acid sequences)

Genome— the complete set of chromosomes derived from one parent, the haploid genome, or the two sets of chromosomes, (e.g., one set from one egg, the other from the sperm), the diploid genome

Genotype— one's genetic makeup or genes

Germinate— develop from a seed into a plant

Glucose— one of the simplest and most important sugars which is the basic transportable form of fuel for living organisms

Golgi apparatus— membranous system close to the cell nucleus that packages protein secretions for export, packages enzymes into lysosomes for cellular use, and modifies proteins destined to become part of cellular membranes

Gram formula weight— an amount of a substance equal in grams to the sum of the atomic weights

Gray matter—neural tissue of the brain and spinal cord that contains nerve-cell bodies as well as nerve fibers; is brownish gray color

Halogens— the column of elements from fluorine to astatine

Heat capacity— the amount of energy needed to raise the temperature of a substance by one degree Celsius or Kelvin

Hemoglobin— oxygen-transporting component of erythrocytes

Hepatic (portal) system— circulation in which the hepatic portal vein carries dissolved nutrients to the liver tissues for processing

Homeostasis— ability of a cell to regulate a stable internal environment by controlling the passage of fluids into and out of the cell

Hormones— steroidal or amino acid-based molecules released to the blood that act as chemical messengers to regulate specific body functions

Hydrocarbon— an organic compound containing only carbon and hydrogen

Hypertension— high blood pressure

Hypertonic solution— solution having a lower water concentration than a solution to which it is compared

Hypotension— low blood pressure

Hypotonic solution— solution having a higher water concentration than a solution to which it is compared

Immune system— a functional system whose components attack foreign substances or prevent their entry into the body

In vitro— in a test tube, glass, or artificial environment

Inert gases— the column of elements from helium to radon; also called noble gases

Inflammation— a nonspecific defensive response of the body to tissue injury, including dilation of blood vessels and an increase in vessel permeability; indicated by redness, heat, swelling, and pain

Inoculation— placement of bacteria onto a culture medium

Inspiration— process of breathing in

Ion— an atom with an electric charge due to gain or loss of electrons

Ionization— adding or subtracting electrons from an atom; alternatively, the dissociation of a solute into ions

Isomers— several molecules with the same composition but different structures

Isotonic solution— a solution with a concentration of nonpenetrating solutes equal to that found in the reference cell

Isotope— a variation of an element characterized by a specific number of neutrons in the nucleus

Joule— a unit of energy equal to 0.239 calorie

Krebs cycle— aerobic metabolic pathway occurring within mitochondria, in which food metabolites are oxidized and CO_2 is liberated, and coenzymes are reduced

Lipid— organic compound formed of carbon, hydrogen, and oxygen (e.g., fats and cholesterol)

Locomotion— voluntary and involuntary movement of body via musculoskeletal system

Lymphatic system— a complex system of thin-walled vessels similar to the blood capillaries, which serve to collect lymph fluid from tissues and organs and to transport the fluid to the venous circulation

Macrophage— protective cell type common in connective tissue, lymphatic tissue, and certain body organs that phagocytizes tissue cells, bacteria, and other foreign debris; important as an antigen-presenter to T cells and B cells in the immune response

Malignant— life threatening; pertains to neoplasms that spread and lead to death; such as cancer

Maltose— a disaccharide or double sugar made of two glucose molecules

Mast cells— immune cells that function to detect foreign substances in the tissue spaces and initiate local inflammatory responses against them; typically found clustered deep to an epithelium or along blood vessels

Mechanical disadvantage (speed lever)— a condition that occurs when the load is far from the fulcrum and the effort is applied near the fulcrum; the effort applied must be greater than the load to be moved

Mechanical energy— the energy directly involved in moving matter (e.g., in cycle riding, the legs provide the mechanical energy that moves the pedals)

Metals— the elements in the middle and left parts of the periodic table, except for hydrogen

Metamorphosis— series of changes that take place as an egg develops into an adult, including the four stages of egg, larva, pupa, and adult

Milliequivalent per liter (mEq/L)— the units used to measure electrolyte concentrations of body fluids; a measure of the number of electrical charges in 1 liter of solution

Mitosis— process of cell duplication, in which two daughter cells receive exactly the same nuclear material as the original cell

Molarity— the number of moles of solute in 1 liter of solution

Mole— an amount of a substance equal in grams to the sum of the atomic weights

Molecule— a group of atoms linked together by covalent bonds

Monosaccharide— a simple sugar that cannot be broken down by hydrolysis (e.g., glucose, fructose, and galactose); building block of carbohydrates

Motor neurons— special nerve cells that transmit impulses to the muscles

Mucous membranes— membranes that form the lining of body cavities open to the exterior (digestive, respiratory, urinary, and reproductive tracts)

Muscle tone— sustained partial contraction of a muscle in response to stretch receptor inputs; keeps the muscle healthy and ready to act

Nephron— structural and functional unit of the kidney; consists of the glomerulus and renal tubule

Neutralization— the chemical reaction of an acid and base to yield a salt and water

Neutron— a heavy subatomic particle with zero change; found in an atomic nucleus

Nonmetals— the elements in the upper-right part of the periodic table, and also hydrogen

Nucleus— the core of an atom, contains protons and neutrons

Nutrient— nourishment; food that promotes growth in living organisms

Nutrition— taking in and breaking down nutrients to be used for metabolism via digestive system

Operant conditioning— a method of using rewards to train an animal to perform tasks that are not innate

Ophthalmic— pertaining to the eye

Optic— pertaining to the eye or vision

Orbital— a classification of the energy level occupied by electrons indicating the probable location of the electrons

Organ— a part of the body formed by two or more tissues and adapted to carry out a specific function (e.g., the stomach)

Organ system— a group of organs that work together to perform a vital body function (e.g., the nervous system)

Organic— refers to compounds based on carbon

Osmosis— movement of water through a semipermeable membrane from an area of greater water concentration to an area of lesser water concentration

Osmotic pressure— force produced by the pressure of water diffusing through a semipermeable membrane; the greater the difference in water concentration on either side of the membrane, the greater the osmotic pressure

Oxidation— a reaction involving the loss of electrons by an element

Oxidation-reduction reaction— a reaction that couples the oxidation (loss of electrons) of one substance with the reduction (gain of electrons) of another substance

Oxygenation— taking in oxygen and expelling carbon dioxide via respiratory system

Pathogen— disease-causing microorganism

Periodic table— display of the elements in order of atomic number with similar elements falling into columns

Peripheral nervous system (PNS)— portion of the nervous system consisting of nerves and ganglia that lie outside of the brain and spinal cord

Peristalsis— wavelike contractions of muscles in tubular organs; motion that forces food through the human digestive organs; means of locomotion in earthworms

Permeability— that property of membranes that permits passage of molecules and ions

pH— a number describing the concentration of hydrogen ions in a solution

Photosynthesis— energy-making reaction in plants; formation of carbohydrates in chlorophyll-containing tissue of plants exposed to light (e.g., carbon dioxide, water, and sunlight are used to produce oxygen, sugar, and energy.)

Phototropism— growth response of plants to light

Pituitary gland— neuroendocrine gland located beneath the brain that serves a variety of functions including regulation of gonads, thyroid, adrenal cortex, lactation, and water balance

Pleural cavities— a subdivision of the thoracic cavity; each houses a lung

Polymer— a large molecule formed by many small molecules linked together in chainlike fashion

Potential energy— stored or inactive energy

Pressure gradient— difference in hydrostatic pressure that drives filtration

Progesterone— hormone partly responsible for preparing the uterus for the fertilized ovum

Prostate gland— accessory reproductive gland, produces one-third of semen volume, including fluids that activate sperm

Proton— a heavy subatomic particle with a positive charge; found in an atomic nucleus

Radioactivity— the emission of subatomic particles from a nucleus

Recessive traits— a trait due to a particular allele that does not manifest itself in the presence of other alleles that generate traits dominant to it; must be present in double dose in order to be expressed

Reduction— a reaction involving the gain of electrons by an element

Regeneration— replacement of destroyed tissue with the same kind of tissue

Regulation— hormonal control of bodily function via endocrine system

Renal— pertaining to the kidney

Reserve air— amount of air that can be forced out of the lungs after normal expiration

Residual air— amount of air left in the lungs after forced expiration

Respiration— reaction in the cells of plants and animals that use oxygen and sugar to produce carbon dioxide, water, and energy

RNA (ribonucleic acid)— genetic material that assists with protein synthesis

Salt— a solid compound composed of both metallic and nonmetallic elements

Saturated— describes a solution that has as much solutes as it can hold at a given temperature.

Scientific method— a series of logically related steps used to gather information in order to solve a problem

Self-duplication— production of offspring via the reproductive system

Semipermeable membrane— a membrane that selectively allows materials to pass through

Sensory neurons— special nerve cells that transmit impulses from a stimulus to a receptor

Sex-linked inheritance— inherited traits determined by genes on the sex chromosomes (e.g., X-linked genes are passed from mother to son; Y-linked genes are passed from father to son.)

Shell— a set of electron orbitals with the same principal quantum number

Skeletal muscle— muscle composed of cylindrical multinucleated cells with striations; skeletal muscle, a voluntary muscle, attaches to the body's skeleton

Solubility— the upper limit to the concentration of a solute

Solubility product— the constant obtained by multiplying the ion concentrations in a saturated solution

Solute— the substance that is dissolved in a solution

Solvent— the host substance of dominant abundance in a solution

Stimulus receptors— sensory organs that respond to stimuli; organs that respond to sight, sound, smell, touch, and taste

Sublimation— the transformation of a solid directly to a gas without an intervening liquid state

Substrate— substance on which an enzyme operates

Tidal air— amount of air involved during normal breathing

Tropism— movement of plants in response to stimuli

Valence— a signed integer describing the combining power of an atom as a real or hypothetical charge

Ventrally— in the front, near the bottom

Vital capacity— maximum volume of air inhaled or exhaled during forced breathing

Section V: English and Language Usage

The English section addresses five principal areas of language arts: punctuation, grammar, sentence structure, contextual words, and spelling. In this section, you will be introduced to the various types of test items common to each of these areas.

This study guide will help you to develop those skills needed to be more prepared for this exam. It takes into consideration the fact that English is an inconsistent language and, grammatically speaking, one of the most difficult. Explanations of grammar usage, sentence structure mechanics, and spelling are presented in the form of lists of rules and examples. This format is thorough, but concise, making it an ideal study tool. Although this study guide is designed to reinforce previously learned material, the simplicity of the format makes it feasible for initial learning to take place.

To facilitate further study and test preparation, explanatory charts compliment the instructional text. Sample test items, complete with answers and explanations, precede a practice test and an answer key.

Punctuation

When you speak, you use the tone of your voice, pauses, hand gestures, facial expressions, and other body language to communicate ideas, feelings, and information. When writing, you must depend on marks of punctuation to assist you in conveying your intended message with maximum clarity.

One objective of the English and Language Usage Exam is to measure your proficiency in written expression. In general, this will entail your reading of passages that contain several grammatical, mechanical, or usage errors that you will cite and/or correct via multiple-choice responses.

If you learn and review the punctuation rules in this section of the English unit, you should be able to spot errors more readily. Schedule some time to review these punctuation rules and their examples.

Marks of Punctuation

Period (.)

1. The period follows a <u>declarative</u> sentence (See *Kinds of Sentences in the Sentence Structure section*).

   Example: Free men should never take their rights for granted.

2. A period follows accepted abbreviations.

   Examples: Mr. Mrs. Dr. M.D. Lieut. Maj. A.D. B.C. etc.

   Note: Abbreviations are used to save time and space. If the piece of writing is to be one of merit then abbreviations should be avoided. When abbreviations are used, consult any standard dictionary for the acceptable forms.

3. A period follows an imperative sentence (See *Kinds of Sentences in the Sentence Structure section*).

   Example: Close the window.

4. A period follows an indirect question.

   Example: He asked his friend why the trains were late.

5. A series of periods (an ellipsis) is used to indicate omission in quoted material. Use three periods at the beginning of a sentence; three in the middle, and four periods at the end of a sentence.

    Example: "...So, now we're taking steps toward improving customer relations."

Comma (,)

1. When words in a series precede the subject of a sentence, they should be offset by commas.

    Example: Red, green, and yellow balloons were chosen for decorations.

2. When a dependent clause precedes an independent clause in a complex sentence, a comma should separate the two.

    Example: If time were gold, some of us could not spend it more foolishly.

3. The introductory words yes and no are set apart by commas.

    Example: Yes, I do plan to attend the meeting.

4. Nonrestrictive phrases and clauses are offset by commas.

    Example: Jack Smith, who studied drama in New York City, is a fine actor.

    Note: If the phrase or clause in question can be excluded from the sentence without greatly changing the meaning, it is classed as nonrestrictive and should be separated with commas.

5. Parenthetical expressions, words of direct address, and appositives are offset by commas.

    Examples: He is, I believe, ready to assume his responsibilities.
    Harry, will you please help me with this problem?
    Mrs. Reiche, our principal, is always doing things for others.
    The weather, a key factor in scheduling the tour, was ideal.

6. Use the comma to separate quoted expressions.

    Examples: He said, "I will be ready on time."
    "The time to leave," she shouted sternly, "is right now!"

7. Words, phrases, or clauses occurring in a series are usually punctuated with commas.

    Examples: Diligence, perseverance, honesty, and self-control, all contribute to success.
    Whenever I become dissatisfied, feeling I have not accomplished a great deal in my life, I pause, count my blessings, and give thanks for the many good things I have been able to do.

    Note: When descriptive words are used that seem to go together, no comma is used.

    Example: The two large bears paused for a few moments to rest.

8. A comma is used to separate city and state.

    Example: He now resides in Denver, Colorado.

9. A comma is used to separate the date from the year.

    Example: She was born August 15, 1991.

10. A comma follows the salutation of a friendly letter.

    Example: Dear Akeem,

Semicolon (;)

1. The semicolon follows an independent clause in a compound sentence if the clauses are not joined by a coordinating conjunction.

    Example: Adelaide sings beautifully; she plays the piano well, too.

    Exception: When the two independent clauses are short or similar, a comma may be used.

    Example: Mark ate the pie, I did not.

    Note: It is usually correct to use the semicolon to separate sentence elements of equal rank. Use a comma preceding the coordinating conjunctions (*and, but, for, yet, so, or,* and *nor*); use a semicolon preceding the conjunctive adverbs, connecting sentence elements of equal rank. Some conjunctive adverbs are as follows: *however, then, therefore, nevertheless, thus, hence, furthermore*, etc.

    Example: The job must be done immediately; therefore, I suggest that we begin now.

2. When sentence elements contain one or more commas, the division between sentence elements should be marked with a semicolon.

    Example: He is bold, obdurate, and lazy; but in spite of these faults, he is honest.

Colon (:)

1. The colon indicates a longer pause than the comma or semicolon. It usually heralds something important that is to follow immediately in the sentence.

    Examples: In dealing with people, keep this in mind: always be master of the situation.
    You must bring the following items: a notebook, a pen, and a pencil.

2. The colon is used to separate the hour from the minutes in expressing time.

    Example: The train will leave at 5:30 p.m.

3. A colon may follow the salutation of a formal letter.

    Example: To whom it may concern:

Dash (–)

1. The dash indicates an interruption or an abrupt change of ideas in a sentence.

    Example: I'm going to leave–you thought I wouldn't, I know–because this time you are in the wrong.

Quotation Marks ("")

1. Enclose the exact words of the speaker within quotation marks.

    Example: Our teacher said, "You should study if you are to succeed."

    Note: Anything taken from a text or other copyrighted source must be enclosed within quotation marks.

2. Use quotation marks to enclose titles of chapters, articles, short poems, short stories, songs, and essays.

   Example: *The two reading selections that I enjoyed most in this month's <u>Reader's</u> <u>Chronicle</u> were the poem "The Fall of the Trees", and the article "Thank a Grandparent".*

   Note: Italicize or underline long works, such as magazines, long poems, newspapers, books, plays, etc. Use quotation marks with short works as noted above (poems, articles, etc.)

3. Use quotation marks to enclose slang words, technical terms, and other expressions that are unusual in Standard English.

   Examples: *She belongs to the "baby boomer" generation.*
   He enjoys "long hair" music.

4. Use single quotation marks when making a quotation within a quotation.

   Example: *"'The curfew tolls the knell of parting day,' is the line I want," said Mr. Song.*

Parentheses ( )

1. Parentheses are used to enclose supplementary or explanatory material which interrupts the main sentence.

   Example: *Mr. Corschwin made the statement publicly (as I knew he would) that he would contribute his services for the good of the organization.*

   Note: Even if the material within the parentheses is a complete declarative or imperative sentence, it is not necessary to use end punctuation if the sentence is short. If the material within the parentheses is a question, then a question mark must be used.

   Example: *Your employer called me on the telephone (did you know?) and inquired why you were not at work.*

Question Mark (?)

1. Use the question mark after a direct question.

   Example: Have you ever heard this musical composition?

   Note: After a polite request (very often in correspondence), use a period.

   Example: Will you please send samples of the material.

Exclamation Mark (!)

1. The exclamation mark is used to express strong feeling.

   Example: Yes! We won the game!

Hyphen (-)

1. Use a hyphen to divide a word at the end of a line when the entire word will not fit on that line. Words of one syllable should not be divided. Words should be divided between syllables and writers should avoid separating a suffix of fewer than three letters from the rest of the word.

   Example: She was not able to place a call to her aunt in Cali-
   fornia.

   Note: If possible, hyphenated words should be divided at the hyphen.

   Example: She planned to begin her trip across the country on the twenty-
   fourth of the month.

2. Use a hyphen with compound numbers from twenty-one to ninety-nine and with fractions used as adjectives.

   Examples: seven hundred and forty-five
   a two-thirds majority

   Note: If the fraction serves as a noun in the sentence, do not use a hyphen.

   Example: There was only one half left.

3. A hyphen is used to form new words beginning with the following prefixes: *self, ex, all, trans,* and *great.* It is also used to join any prefix to a proper adjective or noun. A hyphen is used with the suffix *elect.*

   Examples: ex-player, president-elect, trans-Atlantic, self-confidence, mid-August,
   pre-Renaissance, great-grandfather

4. Hyphenate a compound adjective when it precedes the word it modifies.

   Examples: a well-known artist
   the soft-spoken child

   Note: Do not use a hyphen if one of the modifiers is an adverb ending in *ly.*

   Example: an easily remedied situation

5. Use a hyphen to prevent confusion or awkwardness.

   Examples: re-form the band (prevents confusion with reform)
   re-cover the chair (prevents confusion with recover)

Apostrophe (')

1. An apostrophe is used to form the possessive case or to show ownership of a singular noun. Add an apostrophe and an **s** to the noun.

   Examples: The girl's notebook
   Mark's bike
   The boss's parking space

   Note: When a word of more than one syllable ends in an **s** sound, the singular possessive may be formed by adding the apostrophe only. Omitting the additional *s* eliminates the awkward hiss of repeated **s** sounds.

   Examples: the witness' testimony
   for conscience' sake

2. To form the possessive case or to show ownership of a plural noun that ends in **s**, add only the apostrophe.

   Example: the girls' notebooks

   Note: Plural nouns that do not end in **s** form the possessive or show ownership by adding an apostrophe and an **s** just as singular nouns do.

   Examples: women's health
   children's library

3. Use an apostrophe in certain expressions of time.

   Examples: a week's vacation
   a year's notice

4. Use an apostrophe to pluralize letters, numbers, and words that normally do not have plurals.

   Examples: dot your i's
   grouped by 4's
   no if's or and's about it

5. Use an apostrophe to show omission of letters or numbers as in contractions or dates.

   Examples: can't (contraction for cannot)
   The Class of '05 (2005)

Test Your Knowledge: Punctuation

Using the language rules from the previous section, correct the following sentences. In the right-hand column, identify the rule that was violated. If no errors are found, write *no change* in the right-hand column. Follow this example:

Language Problem(s)

Item 1:	The convention starts tomorrow	* end punctuation
Corrected Sentence:	*The convention starts tomorrow.*	* use of period

Language Problem(s)

Item 2:	The letter was from Mr. D L Stokes.	
Corrected Sentence:		
Item 3:	They shopped for cookies, fruit lunch meat milk and bread.	
Corrected Sentence:		
Item 4:	The weather was hot and dry there was no sign of rain.	
Corrected Sentence:		
Item 5:	When is the train scheduled to arrive.	
Corrected Sentence:		
Item 6:	We went to see Cats on Broadway.	
Corrected Sentence:		
Item 7:	Ed, the car salesman, offered us a great deal.	
Corrected Sentence:		
Item 8:	Look out for the ladder.	
Corrected Sentence:		
Item 9:	The documentary airs at 800 p.m.	
Corrected Sentence:		
Item 10:	He insisted on introducing the contract of course.	
Corrected Sentence:		
Item 11:	I should have chosen the red sports car, said Sharon regretfully.	
Corrected Sentence:		
Item 12:	She asked if he could join them?	
Corrected Sentence:		

Item 13:	The meeting was held April 9 2002.	
Corrected Sentence:		
Item 14:	They wont be here until 10 o'clock	
Corrected Sentence:		
Item 15:	The equipment needed is as follows sleeping bag, flashlight, boots, fishing gear and a hunting knife.	
Corrected Sentence:		
Item 16:	He lives in Dallas Texas.	
Corrected Sentence:		
Item 17:	Watch out for that car	
Corrected Sentence:		
Item 18:	I wanted to go but I had no transportation.	
Corrected Sentence:		
Item 19:	The building which was a firetrap was torn down.	
Corrected Sentence:		
Item 20:	No I did not return her phone call.	
Corrected Sentence:		
Item 21:	Dear Sir:	
Corrected Sentence:		
Item 22:	The cars motor needed repair.	
Corrected Sentence:		
Item 23:	We expect them moment arily.	
Corrected Sentence:		
Item 24:	Ms. Barnes I realized after our meeting is quite capable of managing this position with ease.	
Corrected Sentence:		
Item 25:	There were thirty five people on the guest list.	
Corrected Sentence:		
Item 26:	May I interrupt you for a moment?	
Corrected Sentence:		

Punctuation
Answer Key

Item	Corrected Sentence	Language Problem(s)	Description of Problem(s)
1. The convention starts tomorrow	The convention starts tomorrow.	▪ end punctuation ▪ use of period	tomorrow (a statement is followed by a period)
2. The letter was from Mr. D L Stokes.	The letter was from Mr. D. L. Stokes.	▪ punctuation ▪ use of period	D L (periods after initials omitted)
3. They shopped for cookies, fruit lunch meat milk and bread.	They shopped for cookies, fruit, lunch meat, milk, and bread.	▪ internal punctuation ▪ use of commas	commas omitted (commas in a series)
4. The weather was hot and dry there was no sign of rain.	The weather was hot and dry; there was no sign of rain.	▪ run-on sentences ▪ use of semi-colon	run-on sentence (punctuation omitted)
5. When is the train scheduled to arrive.	When is the train scheduled to arrive?	▪ end punctuation ▪ question mark	question (incorrect end punctuation)
6. We went to see Cats on Broadway.	We went to see *Cats* on Broadway.	▪ Italics or underline	*Cats* (play title in italics required)
7. Ed, the car salesman, offered us a great deal.	Ed, the car salesman, offered us a great deal.	▪ no change	no change
8. Look out for the ladder.	Look out for the ladder!	▪ end punctuation ▪ use of exclamation point	incorrect end punctuation (exclamation)
9. The documentary airs at 800 p.m.	The documentary airs at 8:00 p.m.	▪ punctuation ▪ use of colon	800 (colon omitted)
10. He insisted on introducing the contract of course.	He insisted on introducing the contract (of course). or He insisted on introducing the contract, of course.	▪ punctuation ▪ parenthesis ▪ commas	of course (set off from main idea using parentheses or a comma.)
11. I should have chosen the red sports car, said Sharon regretfully.	"I should have chosen the red sports car," said Sharon regretfully.	▪ punctuation ▪ use of quotation marks	direct quote (quotation marks omitted)
12. She asked if he could join them?	She asked if he could join them.	▪ end punctuation ▪ use of question mark/period	? incorrect end punctuation (indirect question)
13. The meeting was held April 9 2002.	The meeting was held on April 9, 2002.	▪ internal punctuation ▪ use of comma	9 - comma omitted (separate day from year)
14. They wont be here until 10 o'clock	They won't be here until 10 o'clock.	▪ punctuation ▪ use of apostrophe	wont (contraction, apostrophe omitted)

Item	Corrected Sentence	Language Problem(s)	Description of Problem(s)
15. The equipment needed is as follows sleeping bag, flashlight, boots, fishing gear, and a hunting knife.	The equipment needed is as follows: sleeping bag, flashlight, boots, fishing gear, and a hunting knife.	• punctuation • use of colon	as follows (colon needed to precede list)
16. He lives in Dallas Texas.	He lives in Dallas, Texas.	• internal punctuation • use of commas	Dallas Texas (comma between city and state)
17. Watch out for that car	Watch out for that car!	• end punctuation • use of exclamation point	missing end punctuation (exclamatory sentence-needs exclamation point)
18. I wanted to go but I had no transportation.	I wanted to go, but I had no transportation.	• internal punctuation • use of commas	go but (comma between two independent clauses)
19. The building which was a firetrap was torn down.	The building, which was a firetrap, was torn down.	• internal punctuation • use of commas	building…firetrap commas omitted (offset nonessential clauses)
20. No I did not return her phone call.	No, I did not return her phone call.	• internal punctuation • use of commas	no (comma omitted after certain introductory elements)
21. Dear Sir:	Dear Sir:	• no change	no change
22. The cars motor needed repair.	The car's motor needed repair.	• internal punctuation • use of apostrophe	cars (apostrophe omitted, possessive)
23. We expect them moment arily.	We expect them moment-arily.	• punctuation • use of hyphen	moment-arily (syllabication, hypen omitted)
24. Ms. Barnes I realized after our meeting is quite capable of managing this position with ease.	Ms. Barnes–I realized after our meeting–is quite capable of managing this position with ease.	• punctuation • use of dash	Ms. Barnes--I realized after our meeting-- (dash needed, break in thought)
25. There were thirty five people on the guest list.	There were thirty-five people on the guest list.	• punctuation • use of hyphen	thirty five (hyphen needed in two-digit numbers above 20)
26. May I interrupt you for a moment?	May I interrupt you for a moment.	• end punctuation • use of period	incorrect end punctuation (imperative requires a period)

Grammar

Here are some basic rules to help you identify grammatical, mechanical, or usage errors and to provide you with the rationale for their corrections.

Plural Nouns

1. Most nouns are made plural by adding **s** to the singular.

    Examples: book, books; paper, papers; house, houses

2. Add *es* to nouns ending in *ch, sh, s, x,* or *z*

    Examples: rich, riches; brush, brushes; glass, glasses; box, boxes;

    Note: Proper names are generally pluralized by adding *s*. If the proper name ends in *ch, sh, s, x,* or *z*, then add *es*.

    Examples: Charles, Charleses; Perry, Perrys, Walsch, Walsches

3. To make nouns ending in *y* preceded by a consonant plural, change the *y* to *i* and add *es*.

    Examples: study, studies; city, cities; sky, skies

4. For nouns ending in *y* preceded by a vowel, add *s* to form the plural.

    Examples: valley, valleys; trolley, trolleys; turkey, turkeys

5. For most nouns ending in *f* or *fe*, change the *f* to *v* and add *es*

    Examples: calf, calves; elf, elves; half, halves; knife, knives; leaf, leaves; life, lives; loaf, loaves; self, selves; sheaf, sheaves; shelf, shelves; wife, wives; wharf, wharves; wolf, wolves

6. Most nouns ending in *o* preceded by a consonant are made plural by adding *es*.

    Examples: echo, echoes; hero, heroes; mosquito, mosquitoes

7. Other nouns ending in *o* preceded by a vowel become plurals by adding *s*.

    Examples: cameo, cameos; folio, folios; ratio, ratios

    Note: Musical terms add *s* only, whether a vowel or consonant precedes the *o*.

    Examples: banjo, banjos; alto, altos; adagio, adagios

8. Letters, numbers, and symbols become plurals by adding *'s*.

    Examples: Dot your i's and cross your t's.
    There are too many 3's in that column of figures.

9. Compound nouns become plurals by adding **s** and **es** to the main word.

    Examples: brother-in-law, brothers-in-law; go-between, go-betweens; passer-by, passers-by; cross-examination, cross-examinations

10. Some nouns are made plural by changing a vowel or vowels within the word.

    Examples: man, men; foot, feet; goose, geese

11. Some nouns have the same form in the plural as in the singular.

    Examples: Chinese, salmon, sheep, deer

Syllabication: Hyphen Usage

Keep in mind that your best guide is a dictionary; however, the following rules on syllabication should prove helpful.

1. Do not divide words with one syllable.

    Examples: act, blot, debt, ship

2. Use the hyphen when the division of a word occurs at the end of a line. The word should be broken only between syllables.

    Note: Do not carry over to the next line single letters or syllables of two letters.

    Examples: instead of compan-y, break as com-pany;
    instead of final-ly, break as fi-nally

3. Never divide words with four letters. If possible, do not divide words with five or six letters.

4. If a letter of one syllable occurs at the beginning or at the end of a word, do not divide the letter from the rest of the word.

    Example: do not break a-part

5. In words with prefixes, make the division between the prefix and the next letter in the word.

    Examples: ante-chamber, anti-pathy, sub-way, dis-locate

    Note: Avoid making a division if the prefix has only two letters.

    Examples: exclu-sion rather than ex-clusion
    bicip-ital rather than bi-cipital

6. If a word has a suffix, make the division between the suffix and the letter preceding the suffix.

    Examples: accept-able, access-ible, aud-ible, agita-tion, altera-tion

7. If a word has a double consonant, the division should be made between the two consonants. This also includes words that double the final consonant when a termination beginning with a vowel is added.

    Examples: bed-ding, allot-ted, omit-ted

    Note: If a word possesses a double consonant before the suffix is added, make the division after the last consonant.

    Examples: toss-ing, pass-ing, tell-ing

8. Make no divisions in the following combinations of letters: *tch*, latching; *sh*, gusher; *ng*, ringing; *ph*, euphony; *ght*, thoughtful

9. When one letter forms a syllable in a word of three or more syllables, make the division after the single syllable.

    Examples: tele-graphic, medi-cation

10. The suffixes *able, ible; cion, cian; tion, sion; ceed, sede, cede; ance, ence* are not divided.

11. In dividing compound nouns, place the hyphen where the whole word division occurs.

    Examples: brother-in-law, outer-chamber, passer-by

Capitalization

1. Capitalize the first word of every sentence.

    Example: Success in any field of endeavor takes hard work.

    Note: A short sentence enclosed in parentheses within another sentence does not have to begin with a capital letter.

    Example: A teacher's work (it has often been spoken), begins when the dismissal bell rings.

2. Capitalize every line of poetry (although it is the poet's license to disregard the rule in his/her quest for new rhymes and forms).

3. Capitalize the first word in a direct quotation.

    Example: "You will always remember your high school days with fond recollection,"
    Mr. Jackson said.

4. Capitalize the first word of a formal statement or a resolution.

    Example: We are resolved, that all men must live in peace in our time and forever.

5. Capitalize the names of months, days of the week, and holidays.

    Examples: August, September, October; Sunday, Monday, Tuesday; Easter, Christmas,
    Thanksgiving

6. Capitalize geographical names and places.

    Examples: Portland, Maine; White Mountains; South America; Mississippi River

7. Capitalize the words *north, south, east, west* and their compounds when they refer to particular regions. Capitalize nicknames and special names for regions or districts.

    Examples: Western Canada; the South; the West, the Panhandle; the Hub

    Note: Do not capitalize the words **north, south, east, west** when they refer to points of the compass. Do not capitalize these words when they refer to a part of a state.

    Examples: western Kansas; the southern United States

8. Capitalize the names of city streets; parks; buildings; memorials

    Examples: Center Street; Lincoln Park; Chapman Building, Longfellow Monument

    Exceptions: If the street, park, or building is not used as a proper noun, it is lowercase.

    Example: Cheryl and Greg ride their bikes down the street to the park.

9. Capitalize the names of wars, battles, treaties, and important historical events or documents.

    Examples: World War II; Battle of Bulge; the Atlantic Pact

10. Capitalize the names of particular associations; parties, religious groups, etc.

    Examples: Catholic; Protestant; Republican Party; Democratic Party

11. Capitalize proper names and titles of rank or honor.

    Examples: Thomas Wilson, General Mark Clark; Senator Edward Kennedy;
    J. Weston Walsch, M. A.; the Duke of Kent; the Reverend John Thompson;
    Queen Elizabeth; President George W. Bush

12. Do not capitalize the names of the seasons unless they are personified.

    Examples: Of all the seasons, I like summer best.
    Heralded in trumpet blare, comes Spring across the threshold in scented
    frock and maiden hair.

13. Capitalize the names of countries, languages, races, etc., and the names derived from them.

    Examples: Germany, German; America, American; Texas, Texan

14. Capitalize the main words in the titles of books and poems, plays, articles, musical compositions, chapters of books, etc.

    Examples: The Call of the Wild, The Merchant of Venice,
    Growing Poppies in Season, Home on the Range

    Note: It is not customary to capitalize the articles or prepositions when they are used in a title unless they are used at the beginning.

15. Always capitalize the personal pronoun *I*.

16. Capitalize the words *brother, mother, uncle*, or *father* when they are parts of titles or when they can be substituted for proper nouns.

    Example: My Uncle Charles lives in Los Angeles, California. (Uncle is part of the title)
    My aunt lives in Louisiana. (aunt is not part of a title and is not a proper noun)

17. Capitalize the various names of God and the words that refer to a Deity.

    Example: Savior; Messiah; Allah; Shiva; Yaweh; Shango; Osiris; Brahma

PARTS OF SPEECH: This refers to the ways in which words are used in sentences. There are eight different ways words can be used in the English language; therefore, there are eight parts of speech. The parts of speech include the following: verbs, pronouns, adjectives, adverbs, prepositions, conjunctions, and interjections.

Verbs

1. A verb is a word that expresses action or a state of being.

   Examples: smile, jump, shout, laugh, kick, sing, meet, to be, to have

2. Verbs change form to show differences in time.

   *Example: (present tense) We **smile**.*
   *(past tense) We **smiled**.*
   *(future tense) We **will smile**.*

3. Action verbs express physical or mental action.

   *Examples: We **jog**. We **wonder**.*

4. A linking verb links the subject to the predicate adjective or predicate nominative.

   *Example: You **are kind**. (The linking verb **are** links the adjective **kind** to the subject **you**.)*

*Michelle is a doctor. (The linking verb **is** links the predicate nominative **doctor** to the subject **Michelle**.)*

5. Two or more verbs work together in a verb phrase.

   Example: She **will smile**.
   Janna **should have been running**.

6. A verb must agree with its subject in person and number. Keep in mind that if the subject is singular the verb must be singular. If the subject is plural, the verb must be plural.

   Examples: <u>Han</u> **is** a good student. (singular)
   <u>Han</u> and his sister, <u>Mary</u>, **are** good students. (plural)
   <u>He</u> **was** at the movies. (singular)
   <u>They</u> **were** at the movies. (plural)

7. The verb **be** has three present-tense forms: **is**, **are**, and **am**.

   Examples: He **is funny**.
   They **are funny**.
   I **am funny**.

8. The verb **be** has two past tense forms: **was** and **were**.

   Examples: She **was funny**.
   They **were funny**.

9. The past tense form of most verbs ends in **d** or **ed**.

   Example: They **jumped**.

10. Irregular verbs change in spelling to form the past tense and past participle.

   Examples:

Present tense	Past tense	Past participle
go	went	gone
think	thought	thought
lie (to recline)	lay	lain
drink	drank	drunk
write	wrote	written

11. A verb has tenses to indicate the time of an action or statement. Tense is expressed by changes in the form of the verb.

   - **Present Tense** is used mainly to express an action or to help make a statement about something that is happening at the present time.

   *Example: Ms. Gluck **teaches** English.*

   - **Past Tense** is used to express an action or to help make a statement about something that happened in the past.

   *Example: Before she retired, Ms. Gluck **taught** English.*

   - **Future Tense** is used to express an action or to help make a statement about something that will happen in the future. The future tense is formed with <u>will</u> or <u>shall</u>.

*Example: Ms. Gluck **will teach** English next semester.*

- **Present Perfect Tense** is used to express an action or to help make a statement about something that has been completed at some indefinite time in the past. It is formed with <u>have</u> or <u>has</u> and the verb's past participle.

*Example: Ms. Gluck **has taught** English Composition.*

- **Past Perfect Tense** is used to express an action or to help make a statement about something that has been completed in the past and preceded some other past action or event. It is formed with <u>had</u> and the verb's past participle.

*Example: Ms. Gluck **had taught** English prior to this.*

- **Future Perfect Tense** is used to express an action or to help make a statement about something that will be completed in the future before some other action or event. It is formed with <u>will have</u> or <u>shall have</u> and the past participle.

*Example: After this semester, Ms. Gluck **will have taught** every course in the English Department.*

Case of Pronouns

Case shows the relationship of nouns and pronouns, according to their form and position, to other words in a sentence.

1. The following pronouns are used as subjects or subjective complements: ***I, we, you, she, it, they, he.***

    *Example: **He** was the victor in the race. (Subject)*

    Note: Keep in mind that the above-mentioned personal pronouns often follow linking verbs. Some linking verbs are as follows: ***be, am, is, are, was, were, being, been, become, seem, appear, look, feel, taste, grow, remain, smell, sound***, and ***prove***.

    *Example: The winner was **he**. (Predicate nominative)*

2. The following personal pronouns are used as direct objects, objects of prepositions, and indirect objects: ***me, us, him, her, you, it, them***.

    *Example: They gave **me** a watch. (Indirect object)*
    *I spoke to **him**. (Object of a preposition)*
    *They wanted **him** to help us. (Direct object)*

3. Keep in mind that the relative pronoun **who** is used as a subject or as a predicate pronoun.

    *Example: Mr. Jackson is the teacher **who** taught me all I know.*

    Note: In the sentence above, the word ***who*** is used as the subject in the dependent clause, **who taught me all I know**.

4. Keep in mind that the relative pronoun, ***whom,*** is used as an object, or as an object of a prepositional phrase.

    *Example: He is the person of **whom** we spoke. (Object of a preposition)*
    *John was the boy **whom** we asked to help. (Direct object)*

Test Your Knowledge: Grammar

Using the language rules from the previous sections, correct the following sentences. In the right-hand column, identify the rule that was violated. If no errors are found, write *no change* in the right-hand column. Follow this example:

Language Problem(s)

Item 1:	The planes was flying overhead.	* agreement of subject and verb
Corrected Sentence:	*The planes were flying overhead.*	

Language Problem(s)

Item 2:	Each girl was presented with their varsity letter.	
Corrected Sentence:		
Item 3:	Everyone have a favorite dessert.	
Corrected Sentence:		
Item 4:	Several of the members chooses not to vote.	
Corrected Sentence:		
Item 5:	Will you please give Mark and I a ride home?.	
Corrected Sentence:		
Item 6:	Who did you talk to?	
Corrected Sentence:		
Item 7:	My new car has came.	
Corrected Sentence:		
Item 8:	Thelma drunk a cup of coffee.	
Corrected Sentence:		
Item 9:	The boy has laid on the beach all day.	
Corrected Sentence:		
Item 10:	I used to live in New York.	
Corrected Sentence:		
Item 11:	Yesterday, she reports the child missing.	
Corrected Sentence:		
Item 12:	On Saturdays, the cooking is done by me and the laundry is done by my sister.	
Corrected Sentence:		

Item 13:	If I was you, I'd apply for the position.	
Corrected Sentence:		
Item 14:	Nathan had been attending class regular.	
Corrected Sentence:		
Item 15:	She is the most prettiest girl I've ever seen.	
Corrected Sentence:		
Item 16:	I didn't have no time to call.	
Corrected Sentence:		
Item 17:	Asthmatics can't hardly breathe in this humidity.	
Corrected Sentence:		
Item 18:	Evelyn writes good.	
Corrected Sentence:		
Item 19:	"Apparently, there's a monotone between us," chided the choir director.	
Corrected Sentence:		
Item 20:	If he would have run just a little faster, he would have won the race.	
Corrected Sentence:		
Item 21:	They say a woman's home is her castle.	
Corrected Sentence:		
Item 22:	The forecast for tomorrow is sunshine and blue skys.	
Corrected Sentence:		
Item 23:	The food was fit for neither person or beast.	
Corrected Sentence:		
Item 24:	He explained where the concert was at.	
Corrected Sentence:		
Item 25:	Jerry and Raul finishes at 3:00 p.m.	
Corrected Sentence:		
Item 26:	The parents instructed the teens to clean up in their loudest voices.	
Corrected Sentence:		

Grammar
Answer Key

Item	Corrected Sentence	Language Problem(s)	Description of Problem(s)
1. The planes was flying overhead.	The planes were flying overhead.	▪ agreement of subject and verb	planes was (plural subject with singular verb)
2. Each girl was presented with their varsity letter.	Each girl was presented with her varsity letter.	▪ agreement of pronoun and antecedent	Each - their (singular indefinite pronoun, subject – plural antecedent)
3. Everyone have a favorite dessert.	Everyone has a favorite dessert.	▪ singular indefinite pronoun as subject: agreement of subject and verb	Everyone have (singular indefinite pronoun subject – plural verb)
4. Several of the members chooses not to vote	Several of the members choose not to vote.	▪ plural indefinite pronoun as subject: agreement of subject and verb	Several chooses (plural indefinite pronoun subject – singular verb)
5. Will you please give Mark and I a ride home?	Will you please give Mark and me a ride home?	▪ case of pronouns	I (subject pronoun – object pronoun needed)
6. Who did you talk to?	To whom did you talk?	▪ subject and object pronouns used as interrogative pronouns	who (subject pronoun used for an object pronoun)
7. My new car has came.	My new car has come.	▪ principal parts of verbs past participle	has came (incorrect form of past participle)
8. Thelma drunk a cup of coffee.	Thelma drank a cup of coffee.	▪ principal parts of verbs: past participle	drunk (incorrect past tense)
9. The boy has laid on the beach all day.	The boy has lain on the beach all day.	▪ the past participle of lie is lain	has laid (incorrect verb)
10. I used to live in New York.	I used to live in New York.	▪ no change	used to (meaning past residency)
11. Yesterday, she reports the child missing.	Yesterday, she reported the child missing.	▪ tense	reports (present tense verb – past action)
12. On Saturdays, the cooking is done by me and the laundry is done by my sister.	Saturdays, I do the cooking and my sister does the laundry.	▪ use of passive voice	awkward passive voice
13. If I was you, I'd apply for the position.	If I were you, I'd apply for the position.	▪ subjunctive mood	was (contrary to fact – I am *not* you)

Item	Corrected Sentence	Language Problem(s)	Description of Problem(s)
14. Nathan had been attending class regular.	Nathan had been attending class regularly.	▪ correct use of modifiers: adjective and adverb forms	regular (adjective used instead of adverb)
15. She is the most prettiest girl I've ever seen.	She is the prettiest girl I've ever seen.	▪ comparison of adjectives	most prettiest (incorrect superlative)
16. I didn't have no time to call.	I had no time to call.	▪ usage	didn't – no (double negative)
17. Asthmatics can't hardly breathe in this humidity.	Asthmatics can hardly breathe in this humidity.	▪ usage	can't hardly (double negative)
18. Evelyn writes good.	Evelyn writes well.	▪ usage	good (adjective used to modify verb)
19. "Apparently, there's a monotone between us," chided the choir director.	"Apparently, there is a monotone among us," chided the choir director.	▪ usage	between (refers to two)
20. If he would have run just a little faster, he would have won the race.	If he had run just a little faster, he would have won the race.	▪ tense: special problems	would have run; would have won (would have in "if" clause expressing earlier of two past actions)
21. They say a woman's home is her castle.	They say a woman's home is her castle.	▪ no change	woman's (singular noun-possessive)
22. The forecast for tomorrow is sunshine and blue skys.	The forecast for tomorrow is sunshine and blue skies.	▪ plurals of nouns	skys (change y to i add es)
23. The food was fit for neither person or beast.	The food was fit for neither person nor beast.	▪ correlative conjunctions	or (neither . . . nor correlative conjunction pairs)
24. He explained where the concert was at.	He explained where the concert was.	▪ prepositions and prepositional phrases	at (preposition at end of sentence)
25. Jerry and Raul finishes at 3:00 p.m.	Jerry and Raul finish at 3:00 p.m.	▪ agreement of subject and verb	finishes (compound subject requires plural verb)
26. The parents instructed the teens to clean up in their loudest voices.	In their loudest voices, the parents instructed the teens to clean up.	▪ placement of modifiers	in their loudest voices (describes teens instead of parents)

Sentence Structure: Making Sentences

The sentence structure aspect of the English and Language Usage Exam will require you to recognize a complete sentence. A sentence has a subject and a verb/predicate, and it expresses a complete thought. For example: ***Kim drinks only bottled water.*** Kim is the subject and drinks is the predicate.

Test items include sentence fragments and run-on sentences. The sentence fragment is a part of a sentence that does not express a complete thought. Example: ***When she is thirsty.*** You are probably thinking, "Well, what happens when she is thirsty?" The idea initiated is not concluded. The run-on sentence, on the other hand, contains two or more sentences with two or more complete thoughts without correct punctuation. Example: ***Water is her favorite beverage it is a real thirst quencher.***

Some other sentence rules are reviewed below:

Kinds of Sentences

1. A declarative sentence makes a statement. It ends with a period.

   Example: Two amazing football teams played last night.

2. An imperative sentence requests or tells someone to do something. It ends with a period.

   Example: Tell me about the game.

3. An interrogative sentence asks a question. It ends with a question mark.

   Example: Didn't you watch it on television?

4. An exclamatory sentence shows surprise or strong feeling. It ends with an exclamation point.

   Example: It was incredible!

Simple and Compound Sentences

1. A simple sentence contains a complete <u>subject</u> and a complete <u>predicate</u>. It may have a compound subject, a compound predicate, or both.

   Example: <u>Doug</u> <u>dropped</u> the ball.
   <u>Doug</u> and <u>Carl</u> <u>raced</u> for the ball. (Compound subject)
   <u>Doug</u> <u>fell</u> on the ball and <u>recovered</u> it. (Compound predicate)
   <u>Doug</u> and <u>Carl</u> <u>bought</u> and <u>drank</u> two sodas. (Compound subject, Compound predicate)

2. A compound sentence contains at least two simple sentences joined by a conjunction such as ***and***, ***but***, ***or***, ***nor***, ***for***, ***yet***, or ***so***. A comma is used before the conjunction.

   Example: I wanted to leave early, but my boss asked me to stay.

3. A complex sentence contains an independent clause and one or more dependent clauses. An independent clause has a subject and a verb and can stand alone. A dependent clause has a subject and a verb, but it cannot stand by itself and make sense. A dependent clause often begins with a subordinate conjunction such as ***after, as, although, before, because, when, while, that,*** and ***which.***

   Examples: Sarah went to the new health food store. (Independent clause)
   That just opened down the street. (Dependent clause)
   Sarah went to the new health food store that just opened down the street.
   (Complex sentence)

Appositives

An appositive is a noun phrase or clause placed after another noun or pronoun to identify, rename, or explain it. The appositive enhances the understanding of the original noun or pronoun.

Examples: Marilyn, *an amazing cook,* made Mark and me a delicious apple pie.
Bernard, *a true connoisseur of flowers,* won many awards for his tulip bouquets.
The little boy *who just threw his glove to the ground* struck out for the second time.

Note: The first two appositives are set off by commas because they are **nonrestrictive** phrases. **Nonrestrictive** phrases or clauses are those which are not essential to the meaning of the sentence. The third example contains a **restrictive** appositive, which means that the information is necessary to the meaning of the sentence. Do not use commas with restrictive appositives because the information is necessary for the sentence to be clear. The appositive *who just threw his glove to the ground* is needed in the third sentence to identify the boy.

Misplaced Modifiers

Modifiers which have been placed in the incorrect position will make the meaning of a sentence unclear. A modifier should be placed close to the word or phrase it is modifying.

Awkward: Kicking and screaming, the mother changed the baby's diaper. (This is unclear. Is the baby kicking and screaming or the mother?)

Corrected: The mother changed the baby who was kicking and screaming.

Parallel Structure

When two or more parts of a sentence are combined, they must match grammatically in structure. A sentence with grammatically parallel elements will be clear and balanced.

Awkward: Mindy and Will love running, hiking, and to go out to eat in Colorado Springs.

Corrected: In Colorado Springs, Mindy and Will love running, hiking, and eating out.
OR
In Colorado Springs, Mindy and Will love to run, to hike, and to eat out.

Test Your Knowledge: Making Sentences

Create better sentence fluency using the language rules from the previous sections. In the right-hand column, identify the rule that was violated. Follow this example:

		Language Problem(s)
Item 1:	A flaming sun setting beyond the hill.	* sentence fragments
Corrected Sentence:	*A flaming sun was setting beyond the hill.*	

		Language Problem(s)
Item 2:	Marsha scolded the boy. calling him an ungrateful brat.	
Corrected Sentence:		
Item 3:	Chang and I often disagree, although I always respect his opinions.	
Corrected Sentence:		
Item 4:	They moved into the house a small three-room cottage.	
Corrected Sentence:		
Item 5:	She was late for work today, she overslept again.	
Corrected Sentence:		
Item 6:	When the car hit the pole, it snapped in half.	
Corrected Sentence:		
Item 7:	During the summer, I usually like swimming and to water ski.	
Corrected Sentence:		
Item 8:	The administrator adjourned the meeting rapping the gavel.	
Corrected Sentence:		
Item 9:	Mr. Thomas was fired from Washington High because so many students failed the exam. This was unfortunate.	
Corrected Sentence:		
Item 10:	I had a chemistry test coming up on Monday. I had studied for the test. I was apprehensive.	
Corrected Sentence:		
Item 11:	The meeting lasted all day, and nothing was accomplished.	
Corrected Sentence:		

Item 12:	Every time the committee met with the Jones family, the media attacked them.	
Corrected Sentence:		
Item 13:	The architects visited several sites for a location for the community center. The architects turned them all down. The reason the architects turned them all down was because of drainage problems.	
Corrected Sentence:		

Making Sentences
Answer Key

Item	Corrected Sentence	Language Problem(s)	Description of Problem(s)
1. A flaming sun setting beyond the hill.	A flaming sun was setting beyond the hill.	■ sentence fragments	setting (no verb)
2. Marsha scolded the boy. calling him an ungrateful brat.	Marsha scolded the boy calling him an ungrateful brat.	■ phrase fragments	calling him an ungrateful brat (no subject and verb)
3. Chang and I often disagree, although I always respect his opinions.	Although Chang and I often disagree, I always respect his opinions.	■ subordinate ideas order	Although I always respect his opinions (position of secondary idea)
4. They moved into the house a small three-room cottage.	They moved into the house, a small three-room cottage.	■ appositive fragment	A small three-room cottage (appositive not included in sentence of which it is a part)
5. She was late for work today, she overslept again.	She was late for work today because she overslept again.	■ run-on sentences	She was late for work today. She overslept again (two independent clauses improperly joined)
6. When the car hit the pole, it snapped in half.	When the car hit it, the pole snapped in half.	■ ambiguous/unclear reference	it (the car or the pole)
7. During the summer, I usually like swimming and to water ski.	During the summer, I usually like swimming and water skiing.	■ parallel structure	swimming and to water ski (gerund paired with infinitive)
8. The administrator adjourned the meeting rapping the gavel.	Rapping the gavel, the administrator adjourned the meeting.	■ placement of modifiers	rapping the gavel (Was the gavel rapped by the meeting?)
9. Mr. Thomas was fired from Washington High because so many students failed the exam. This was unfortunate.	It is unfortunate Mr. Thomas was fired from Washington High because so many students failed the exam.	■ general/unclear reference	This (a reference to which idea)
10. I had a chemistry test coming up on Monday. I had studied for the test. I was apprehensive.	The teacher had scheduled a chemistry test for Monday. Although I had studied, I was still apprehensive.	■ sentence variety	I had I had I was (subject-verb order repeated)

Item	Corrected Sentence	Language Problem(s)	Description of Problem(s)
11. The meeting lasted all day, and nothing was accomplished.	The meeting lasted all day, however nothing was accomplished.	▪ faulty coordination	and (two ideas of unequal importance joined by a coordinating conjunction)
12. Every time the committee met with the Jones family, the media attacked them.	Every time the committee met with the Jones family, the media attacked the members of the committee.	▪ weak/clear reference	them (whom?)
13. The architects visited several sites for a location for the community center. The architects turned them all down. The reason the architects turned them all down was because of drainage problems.	The architects visited several sites for a location for a community center. They turned them all down because of drainage problems.	▪ ineffective sentence fluency	▪ sentences too short to be effective ▪ sentence variety needed

Contextual Words

Questions in this section test your ability to use context clues to determine the missing word. Context clues are other words surrounding the unfamiliar word.

1. Choose the word that best fits the blank:

    Marilyn entered the room and quickly opened the window. The room reeked with an unidentifiable _____.
      A. *stencil*
      B. *fragrance*
      C. *aroma*
      D. *stench*

The most important clues in the sample test item above are: **reek** and **quickly opened the window**. **Reeked** implies a smell, and **quickly opened the window** suggests that the smell was unpleasant. Aromas and fragrances are not necessarily unpleasant, but stench is. **Stencil** is a distractor that simply shares the same first 4 letters with **stench**.

Other samples of context clues test items follow:

2. Choose the meaning of the underlined word in the sentence.

    Dervin's childish behavior is <u>reminiscent</u> of days gone by when he would throw temper tantrums daily at his nursery school.
      A. *remiss*
      B. *reluctant*
      C. *remindful*
      D. *relevant*

    Note: Context clue is the phrase "of days gone by". Think: memories of days gone by.

    Answer: C.

3. Read the sentence below. Then choose the sentence in which the underlined word is used in the same way.

    The bow of the ship <u>pitched</u> in the heavy seas.

      A. *Ross <u>pitched</u> all nine innings.*
      B. *The scouts <u>pitched</u> their tent at the campsite.*
      C. *The roof was <u>pitched</u> at an angle to allow water to run toward the gutters.*
      D. *The people <u>pitched</u> to and fro as the subway train rumbled down the track.*

    Note: This kind of test item uses multiple-meaning words, or words with many different meanings. Think: A ship in heavy seas would surely rock back and forth; so do people who stand while riding a subway train.

    Answer: D.

Let's examine the eight kinds of clues that will help you zero in on the meaning of an unfamiliar word.

1. **DEFINITION:** In his woodworking, he used a type of file known as a <u>rasp</u>.

2. **DESCRIPTION**: Allen is a <u>malcontent</u>; he is constantly changing jobs, moving to different apartments, and trading in cars. He complains and expresses his dissatisfaction with every aspect of life.

3. **EXAMPLES**: The menu listed such <u>delicacies</u> as frog legs, octopus, and chocolate-flavored worms.

4. **SYNONYMS**: The <u>ophthalmologist</u>, or eye doctor, prescribed eyedrops.

5. **ANTONYMS**: Unlike the sophisticated life in the city, Scottsville was a <u>quaint</u> existence.

6. **COMPARISON**: Elliott is wealthy and generous as is his <u>philanthropist</u> father.

7. **CONTRAST**: The instructor would often <u>deviate</u> from the topic, rather than remain focused on the subject introduced at the beginning of the lecture.

8. **EXPLANATION OF SITUATION**: He was awarded a degree <u>posthumously</u>; he died a month before graduation.

Remember, you may not find the context clues in the same sentence as the underlined word or blank. Read the sentences before and after that sentence carefully. Try to figure out the meaning of the word before reading the answer choices. Read the sentence repeatedly, inserting a different answer choice each time. Be careful of words that fit the sentence but do not really fit the context clues. If the question features a multiple-meaning word, make sure the word you choose is the same part of speech as the one in the test sentence.

The chart at the end of this section will help you to pinpoint contextual clues. Use it as a study strategy as you prep for the test.

Test Your Knowledge: Contextual Words

In each of the following sentences, decipher the meaning of the underlined word based on clues provided in the sentence. In the right-hand column, identify the context clues.

Context Clue(s)

Item 1:	He was awarded the degree in <u>absentia</u>; he was unable to attend graduation.	"unable to attend"
Definition:	*State of not being present or in attendance*	

Context Clue(s)

Item 2:	She had <u>surmounted</u> many challenges, but she would not overcome this one.	
Definition:		
Item 3:	Much to our surprise, Don was not <u>hostile</u>, but warm and friendly.	
Definition:		
Item 4:	John's <u>culinary</u> delights lined the buffet table; there were chicken Kiev, shrimp Creole, and pilaf.	
Definition:		
Item 5:	The old Victorian mansion was <u>tenebrous</u> until the caretaker opened the drapes, letting in light.	
Definition:		
Item 6:	The <u>kayak</u>, a canoe made of seal skin, floated near the fishing pier.	
Definition:		
Item 7:	Like the <u>waning</u> moon, hope diminished with each passing day.	
Definition:		
Item 8:	There were no sidewalks; <u>pedestrians</u> had to be careful to avoid cars.	
Definition:		
Item 9:	The guide <u>reiterated</u> the possibility of danger to each person as he or she entered the bus.	
Definition:		
Item 10:	Many movie stars attend the <u>premiere</u>, or first showing of a movie.	
Definition:		
Item 11:	Mr. Giles is <u>cantankerous</u>. He quarrels and starts arguments with everyone.	
Definition:		
Item 12:	Scrubbing floors, washing dishes, and sifting garbage are just a few of the <u>menial</u> jobs he worked.	
Definition:		
Item 13:	While Sharon was less than enchanted with the show, Karen sat starry-eyed and <u>mesmerized</u>.	
Definition:		

Test Your Knowledge: Contextual Words
Answer Key

Items	Definition	Context Clues	Clue Type
1. He was awarded the degree in <u>absentia</u>; he was unable to attend graduation.	state of not being present or in attendance	▪ "unable to attend"	explanation of situation
2. She had <u>surmounted</u> many challenges, but she would not overcome this one.	rise above, overcome, surpass	▪ "overcome"	synonym
3. Much to our surprise, Don was not <u>hostile</u>, but warm and friendly.	unfriendly	▪ "warm and friendly"	antonym
4. John's <u>culinary</u> delights lined the buffet table; there were chicken Kiev, shrimp Creole, and pilaf.	of or having to do with cooking or the kitchen	▪ "buffet table", "chicken Kiev", "shrimp Creole", "pilaf"	examples
5. The old Victorian mansion was <u>tenebrous</u> until the caretaker opened the drapes, letting in light.	dark, gloomy, obscure	▪ "opened the drapes, letting in the light"	contrast
6. The kayak, a canoe made of seal skin, floated near the fishing pier.	a canoe	▪ "a canoe made of seal skin"	definition
7. Like the <u>waning</u> moon, hope diminished with each passing day.	lessening, becoming smaller	▪ "diminished"	comparison
8. There were no sidewalks; <u>pedestrians</u> had to be careful to avoid cars.	people on foot	▪ "sidewalks"	explanation of situation
9. The guide <u>reiterated</u> the possibility of danger to each person as he or she entered the bus.	to repeat or say over and over again	▪ "to each person"	explanation of situation
10. Many movie stars attend the <u>premiere</u>, or first showing of a movie.	first performance	▪ "first showing"	definition
11. Mr. Giles is <u>cantankerous</u>. He quarrels and starts arguments with everyone.	ill natured, quarrelsome	▪ "quarrels", "starts arguments"	description
12. Scrubbing floors, washing dishes and sifting garbage are just a few of the <u>menial</u> jobs he worked.	related to domestic servant, of lower means	▪ "scrubbing floors", "washing dishes", "sifting garbage"	examples
13. While Sharon was less than enchanted with the show, Karen sat starry-eyed and <u>mesmerized</u>.	subjected to spell-binding influence, hypnotize	▪ "less than enchanted", "while"	contrast

Spelling

Spelling poses considerable concern for many people. This may be due to the numerous inconsistencies in English spelling, or perhaps to common mispronunciation of many words. For instance, we tend to slur some words to the point of omitting syllables and hence a letter or two. We say "accidently" instead of accident**al**ly. The **al** is left out of our pronunciation of the word, which often translates into a spelling error as well.

The spelling test asks you to choose the correct spelling of a word. Your first step is to eliminate the answers that are obviously misspelled or that you <u>know</u> are incorrect. Then examine the remaining choices and select the one that appears most familiar. Apply extreme caution when faced with choices that include homonyms or homophones; these words sound alike but are generally spelled differently and have different meanings.

It will help if you know some basic spelling rules. Examine the following spelling rules as well as the lists of Troublesome and Commonly Misspelled Words and Commonly Confused Words that appear at the end of this section.

(Incidentally, mi<u>s</u>pelled is mi**ss**pelled if it doesn't have a double **s.**)

SPELLING RULES

1. "ie" and "ei" words: **i** before **e,** except after **c**—or when sounded like **a** as in the words **neighbor** and **weigh**.

   Exceptions: either, neither, seize, weird, leisure, inveigle, ancient, species, height, protein, foreign

Examples:	niece	reign	conceive
	ceiling	siege	weigh
	neighbor	receipt	friend
	believe	sleigh	receive
	conceit	grievous	veil

2. Suffixes to words ending in "e": If a word ends in silent **e**, retain the letter **e** if the added suffix begins with a consonant. Drop the letter **e** if the suffix begins with a vowel.

   Exceptions: Retain the letter **e** with words that end in **ce** or **ge** when the suffix **able** or **ous** is added.

Examples:	hate	hateful	age	aging
	enforce	enforcing	awe	awesome
	true	truism	change	changeable

Other Exceptions:	abridge	abridgment	due	duly
	acknowledge	acknowledgment	judge	judgment
	argue	argument	true	truly

3. Words ending in "y": Generally, words that end with **y** preceded by a vowel retain the **y** when any suffix is added. If the final **y** is preceded by a consonant, change the **y** to **i** before any suffix except one beginning with the letter **i**.

Examples:	annoy	annoyance	country	countrified
	buy	buyer	carry	carriage
	enjoy	enjoyable	glory	glorious
	convey	conveyance	hurry	hurried
	delay	delayed	magnify	magnificent
	employ	employer	necessary	necessarily
	survey	surveyor	satisfy	satisfied
	pay	payable	victory	victorious
	journey	journeyed		

4. Words ending in a consonant: For single-syllable words, multi-syllable words accented on the last syllable, words ending in one consonant, and words preceded by one vowel, double the final consonant before adding a suffix beginning with a vowel.

Example:	bag	baggage	allot	allotted
	bar	barred	control	controller
	bed	bedding	corral	corralled
	get	getting	forget	forgettable
	rub	rubbed	occur	occurrence
	run	running	prefer	preferred
	sag	sagging	excel	excellence
	shut	shutting	omit	omitted
	sit	sitting	refer	referred
			compel	compelling

5. Words ending in "c": If a word ends in **c** and a suffix beginning with **e**, **i**, or **y** is added, the letter **k** is usually inserted following the letter **c**.

Examples:	colic	colicky
	frolic	frolicked
	mimic	mimicked
	panic	panicky
	shellac	shellacked

6. Words ending in "ceed," "sede," and "cede"

In English there are three words that end in **ceed**, and one word that ends in **sede**. Other words with the same sound end in **cede**.

Examples:	exceed	supersede	accede
	proceed		antecede
	succeed		concede
			intercede
			recede

7. Words ending in "ise" and "ize": The following words are spelled with the **ise** ending. All other words with the same sound are spelled with the **ize** ending.

Examples:	advertise	devise	premise
	advise	disguise	reprise
	arise	enterprise	revise
	chastise	excise	supervise
	circumcise	exercise	surmise
	comprise	franchise	surprise
	compromise	improvise	despise
	demise	incise	merchandise

8. Words ending in "able" or "ible": There is no definite rule for words ending in **able** or **ible**.

Examples:	acceptable	innumerable	accessible
	available	miserable	audible
	charitable	probable	contemptible
	dependable	profitable	convertible
	durable	notable	divisible

9. Words ending in "ance" or "ence": If the suffix is preceded by the letter **c** having the sound of **s**, or if the suffix is preceded by the letter **g** having the sound of **j**, the suffixes **ence**, **ency**, and **ent** are used. If the suffix is preceded by the letter **c** having the sound of the letter **k**, or if the suffix is preceded by the letter **g** having a hard sound, then the suffixes should be **ance**, **ancy**, or **ant**. If the suffix is preceded by a letter other than the letter **c**, and you are in doubt, consult a dictionary.

Examples:	significance	significant	negligence
	extravagance	vacant	beneficence
	elegant	absence	indigence
		innocence	

10. Words ending in "er," "or," and "ar":

Example:	admirer	bachelor	altar
	counter	collector	beggar
	customer	conductor	cedar
	designer	distributor	collar
	diameter	elevator	grammar
	disorder	inferior	guitar
	earlier	inspector	mortar
	founder	inventor	similar
	happier	junior	peculiar
		odor	vicar

11. Words ending in "tion," "sion," or "cian":

Examples:	agitation	admission	magician
	alteration	allusion	musician
	demonstration	collision	physician
	indication	confusion	politician
	nomination	discussion	technician

Troublesome and Commonly Misspelled Words

Group 1

1. accidentally
2. accommodate
3. accompanied
4. achieved
5. address
6. aggravate
7. anxiety
8. barren
9. believe
10. ceiling
11. confident
12. course
13. disappear
14. disappoint
15. dissipate
16. efficiency
17. emphasize
18. exaggerate
19. exceed
20. fiery
21. finally
22. financial
23. forehead
24. foreign
25. forfeit
26. grief
27. handkerchief
28. hurriedly
29. hypocrisy
30. imminent
31. incidentally
32. innocence
33. intentionally
34. interest
35. legitimate
36. likely
37. manual
38. mattress
39. misspell
40. niece
41. occasion
42. organization
43. parallel
44. piece
45. psychiatrist
46. psychology
47. receive
48. religious
49. severely
50. villain

Group 2

1. arctic
2. auxiliary
3. business
4. candidate
5. characteristic
6. chauffeur
7. colonel
8. column
9. cylinder
10. environment
11. especially
12. exhaust
13. exhilaration
14. February
15. foremost
16. ghost
17. government
18. grievous
19. hygiene
20. intercede
21. leisure
22. library
23. lightning
24. literature
25. mathematics
26. medicine
27. mortgage
28. muscle
29. notoriety
30. optimistic
31. pamphlet
32. parliament
33. physically
34. physician
35. prairie
36. prejudice
37. pronunciation
38. recede
39. recognize
40. reign
41. rhetoric
42. rhythm
43. schedule
44. sentinel
45. soliloquy
46. sophomore
47. studying
48. surprise
49. twelfth
50. Wednesday

Group 3

1. apparent
2. appearance
3. attendance
4. beggar
5. brilliant
6. calendar
7. carriage
8. conqueror
9. contemptible
10. coolly
11. descent
12. desirable
13. dictionary
14. disastrous
15. eligible
16. equivalent
17. existence
18. familiar
19. grammar
20. guidance
21. hindrance
22. hoping
23. imaginary
24. incredible
25. indigestible
26. indispensable
27. inevitable
28. influential
29. irresistible
30. liable
31. marriage
32. momentous
33. naturally
34. nickel
35. noticeable
36. nucleus
37. obedience
38. outrageous
39. pageant
40. permissible
41. perseverance
42. persistent
43. pleasant
44. possible
45. prevalent
46. resistance
47. similar
48. strenuous
49. vengeance
50. vigilance

Group 4

1. allot
2. allotted
3. barbarian
4. barbarous
5. beneficial
6. benefited
7. changeable
8. changing
9. commit
10. committed
11. committee
12. comparative
13. comparatively
14. comparison
15. compel
16. compelled
17. competent
18. competition
19. compulsion
20. conceive
21. conceivable
22. conception
23. conscience
24. conscientious
25. conscious
26. courteous
27. courtesy
28. deceit
29. deceive
30. deception
31. decide
32. decision
33. defer
34. deference
35. deferred
36. describe
37. description
38. device
39. devise
40. discuss
41. discussion
42. dissatisfied
43. dissatisfy
44. equip
45. equipment
46. equipped
47. excel
48. excellent
49. explain
50. explanation

Group 5

1. hesitancy
2. hesitate
3. instance
4. instant
5. intellectual
6. intelligence
7. intelligent
8. intelligible
9. maintain
10. maintenance
11. miniature
12. minute
13. ninetieth
14. ninety
15. ninth
16. obligation
17. oblige
18. obliged
19. occur
20. occurred
21. occurrence
22. omission
23. omit
24. omitted
25. procedure
26. proceed
27. picnic
28. picnicking
29. possess
30. possession
31. precede
32. precedence
33. preceding
34. prefer
35. preference
36. preferred
37. rally
38. realize
39. refer
40. reference
41. referred
42. repeat
43. repetition
44. transfer
45. transferred
46. tried
47. tries
48. try
49. writing
50. written

Group 6

1. obstacle
2. operate
3. opinion
4. pastime
5. persuade
6. piece
7. politician
8. practically
9. presence
10. processor
11. propeller
12. quantity
13. recommend
14. region
15. relieve
16. representative
17. reservoir
18. restaurant
19. ridiculous
20. sacrifice
21. sacrilegious
22. safety
23. salary
24. scarcely
25. science
26. secretary
27. seize
28. separate
29. shriek
30. siege
31. similar
32. suffrage
33. supersede
34. suppress
35. syllable
36. symmetry
37. temperament
38. temperature
39. tendency
40. tournament
41. tragedy
42. truly
43. tyranny
44. unanimous
45. unusual
46. usage
47. valuable
48. wholly
49. yoke
50. yolk

Group 7

1. accept
2. across
3. aisle
4. all right
5. amateur
6. annual
7. appropriate
8. argument
9. arrangement
10. association
11. awkward
12. bachelor
13. biscuit
14. cafeteria
15. career
16. cemetery
17. completely
18. convenient
19. cruelty
20. curiosity
21. definite
22. desperate
23. diphtheria
24. discipline
25. disease
26. distribute
27. dormitories
28. drudgery
29. eighth
30. eliminate
31. ecstasy
32. eminent
33. enemy
34. except
35. exercise
36. extraordinary
37. fascinate
38. fraternity
39. furniture
40. grandeur
41. height
42. imitation
43. interest
44. livelihood
45. loneliness
46. magazine
47. material
48. messenger
49. mischievous

Commonly Confused Words

affect: to influence
effect: noun: the result
      verb: to produce

ascent: climbing, a way sloping up
assent: agreement, to agree

all ready: everyone is ready
already: by this time

all together: as a group
altogether: entirely, completely

altar: a structure used in worship
alter: to change

breath: air taken into the lungs
breathe: to exhale and inhale

capital: chief; leading or governing city; wealth, resources
capitol: a building that houses the state or national lawmakers

cite: to use as an example, to quote
site: location

clothes: wearing apparel
cloths: two or more pieces of cloth

complement: that which completes; to supply a lack
compliment: praise, flattering remark; to praise

corps: a military group or unit
corpse: a dead body

council: an assembly of lawmakers
counsel: advice; one who advises; to give advice

dairy: a factory or farm engaged in milk production
diary: a daily record of experiences

descent: a way sloping down
dissent: disagreement; to disagree

dining: eating
dinning: making a continuing noise

dying: ceasing to live
dyeing: process of coloring fabrics

forth: forward in place or space, onward in time
fourth: the ordinal equivalent of the number four

loose: free from bonds
lose: to suffer a loss

personal: pertaining to a particular person; individual
personnel: body of persons employed in same work or service

principal: chief, most important; a school official; a capital sum (as distinguished from interest or profit)
principle: a belief; rule of conduct or thought

respectfully: with respect
respectively: in order, in turn

stationary: not moving
stationery: writing paper

their: possessive form of they
they're: contraction of they are
there: adverb of place

to: a preposition
too: an adverb which indicates degree
two: the number

whose: possessive form of who
who's: contraction of who is

your: possessive form of you
you're: contraction of you are

Final Prep

If you have kept to your study plan, you should be ready for a final review before attempting the practice test. Follow these suggestions for a more meaningful review.

Use the four study sections in this unit to guide you in your review. A basic grammar textbook might be helpful if you feel you need further clarification on a particular grammar, usage, or mechanics concept.

Spend some time looking over the spelling lists. Highlight words that you know have been a problem for you.

Adjust your thinking mode to that of an editor. Review the checklist below and be aware of the kinds of errors you are looking for.

- ____ Sentences begin with capital letters.
- ____ Sentences have correct ending punctuation.
- ____ Sentences are complete.
- ____ Paragraphs are indented.
- ____ Commas are used in compound sentences which are connected by a coordinating conjunction.
- ____ Commas are used for listing items in a series.
- ____ Quotation marks are used correctly.
- ____ Apostrophes are used correctly for contractions.
- ____ Spelling is correct.
- ____ Unnecessary words, phrases, and sentences have been eliminated.
- ____ Use of common homonyms (there, their, they're; to, too, two; your, you're) are correct.
- ____ Verb tenses are correct.
- ____ Subjects and predicates agree.
- ____ Pronouns agree with the nouns they replace.
- ____ Apostrophes are used correctly for possessive nouns.
- ____ Proper nouns and adjectives are capitalized.
- ____ Colons are used correctly.
- ____ Semicolons are used correctly.
- ____ Underlining (or italics) is used correctly.
- ____ Parentheses are used correctly.
- ____ Dashes are used correctly.

Good Luck!

Test Information

The English examination you are about to take is multiple-choice with only one correct answer per item. Photocopy the answer sheet on this page to record your choices. Circle the correct answers on your answer sheet for each test item. When you have completed the entire test, you may check your answers with those listed on the answer key that follows the English and Language Usage Practice Test.

English and Language Usage Practice Test
Answer Sheet

Sample Test Items

1. **a**   b   c   d
2. a   b   **c**   d

1.	a	b	c	d		29.	a	b	c	d
2.	a	b	c	d		30.	a	b	c	d
3.	a	b	c	d		31.	a	b	c	d
4.	a	b	c	d		32.	a	b	c	d
5.	a	b	c	d		33.	a	b	c	d
6.	a	b	c	d		34.	a	b	c	d
7.	a	b	c	d		35.	a	b	c	d
8.	a	b	c	d		36.	a	b	c	d
9.	a	b	c	d		37.	a	b	c	d
10.	a	b	c	d		38.	a	b	c	d
11.	a	b	c	d		39.	a	b	c	d
12.	a	b	c	d		40.	a	b	c	d
13.	a	b	c	d		41.	a	b	c	d
14.	a	b	c	d		42.	a	b	c	d
15.	a	b	c	d		43.	a	b	c	d
16.	a	b	c	d		44.	a	b	c	d
17.	a	b	c	d		45.	a	b	c	d
18.	a	b	c	d		46.	a	b	c	d
19.	a	b	c	d		47.	a	b	c	d
20.	a	b	c	d		48.	a	b	c	d
21.	a	b	c	d		49.	a	b	c	d
22.	a	b	c	d		50.	a	b	c	d
23.	a	b	c	d		51.	a	b	c	d
24.	a	b	c	d		52.	a	b	c	d
25.	a	b	c	d		53.	a	b	c	d
26.	a	b	c	d		54.	a	b	c	d
27.	a	b	c	d		55.	a	b	c	d
28.	a	b	c	d						

English and Language Usage

Read each sample question below and note the correct answer shown on the answer sheet.

SAMPLES

1. The children play together.
   a. No change
   b. played
   c. is playing
   d. plays

2. Which word means the opposite of **synthetic**?
   a. fabricated
   b. expensive
   c. natural
   d. fake

Questions 1 through 30 pertain to the following passage. Portions of the passage are underlined; each underlined portion is identified with a question or item number. Determine if the underlined part uses correct grammar and punctuation. If it is correct, mark option A, "no change," as your answer. Otherwise, choose the option that you think makes the underlined portion correct.

Even after five years, Lisa Lambert of Fontana, California, paused (1) <u>every time</u> she saw a Lhasa Apso, hoping to discover one blue eye and one brown. But each time her heart (2) <u>sunk</u>. "It's not (3) <u>Sparky,</u>" the (4) <u>38 year old</u> mother of (5) <u>too</u> would sigh sadly.

No one in her family could forget the last time they saw (6) <u>there</u> dog. They (7) <u>were watching</u> July 4th fireworks on television when, spooked by loud (8) <u>pops;</u> the pooch bolted for the open front door and disappeared (9)<u>.</u> The Lamberts were devastated.

From the day they adopted (10) <u>her</u> the odd-eyed dog (11) <u>had gave</u> them all her love. Now she was gone. The Lamberts searched the (12) <u>neighborhood</u> and posted fliers. But no one (13) <u>responds</u>. "When is Sparky coming (14) <u>home,</u>" eight-year-old Susan sadly asked her older brother Robert. But Robert (15) <u>couldn't</u> answer.

Somehow the Lamberts didn't (16) <u>loose</u> hope. "I feel she's out there," Lisa told her husband, Walter. But soon their hope wore thin.

Five years later, Walter (17) <u>recieved</u> a call from a (18) <u>near by</u> animal shelter saying that (19) <u>"they had his dog!"</u> "Could it be?" Lisa's heart pounded as she and Walter rushed over. But when Lisa (20) <u>in the tiny cage looked,</u> she collapsed with a feeling of true (21) <u>elation</u>. (22) <u>Skinny with matted hair</u>. It couldn't be! But when she lifted the dog's face, there was one blue eye and one brown! (23) <u>"Sparky"</u> Lisa cried.

The animal control officer explained (24) they'd been hours away from (25) euphanizing the badly (26) dehydrated dog when they scanned her and discovered a microchip with a tracking number (27) linking her to the Lamberts. The family (28) had the ID chip implanted when Sparky was first adopted.

Sparky had been found just in time. "She hung on for you," the vet (29) marveled.

(30) "It's a miracle!" shouted Lisa.

1. a. no change
    b. everytime
    c. ev'ry time
    d. ever

2. a. no change
    b. sinked
    c. had sunk
    d. sank

3. a. no change
    b. :
    c. ,
    d. ?

4. a. no change
    b. 38-year-old
    c. 38-year old
    d. 38 year-old

5. a. no change
    b. two
    c. to
    d. too

6. a. no change
    b. their
    c. they're
    d. thier

7. a. no change
    b. are watching
    c. watched
    d. had been watching

8. a. no change
    b. :
    c. ,
    d. .

9. a. no change
    b. ?
    c. ,
    d. :

10. a. no change
    b. , her
    c. she
    d. her,

11. a. no change
    b. had given
    c. would give
    d. would have given

12. a. no change
    b. nieghborhood
    c. neighberhood
    d. nayborhood

13. a. no change
    b. has respond
    c. responded
    d. was going to respond

14. a. no change
    b. –
    c. ?
    d. .

15. a. no change
    b. could'nt
    c. coul'dnt
    d. couldno't

16. a. no change
    b. loss
    c. lost
    d. lose

17. a. no change
    b. received
    c. receives
    d. would receive

18. a. no change
    b. neir by
    c. nierby
    d. nearby

19. a. no change
    b. they had had his dog.
    c. they had his dog!
    d. "that they had had his dog"

20. Which phrase would best replace
    the phrase - in the tiny cage looked.?
    a. looked in the cage, tiny,
    b. tiny, looked in the cage,
    c. looked in the tiny cage,
    d. caged and tiny looked in

21. What is a synonym for elation?
    a. sorrow
    b. joy
    c. fainted
    d. fatigue

22. Which option would best replace the
    phrase - skinny with matted hair?
    a. With matted hair and skinny.
    b. Inside, with skinny and matted
       hair
    c. The dog in the cage was skinny
       with matted hair.
    d. Matted hair, she was skinny.

23. a. no change
    b. "Sparky!"
    c. "Sparky?"
    d. "Sparky."

24. a. no change
    b. they would
    c. they could
    d. they would have been

25. a. no change
    b. euthanizing
    c. euphinizing
    d. euphasizing

26. a. no change
    b. dehydration
    c. dehidrated
    d. dehydrate

27. a. no change
    b. linking her for the Lamberts.
    c. linking her too the Lamberts
    d. linking her as the Lamberts

28. a. no change
    b. has had
    c. had had
    d. is having

29. a. no change
    b. marvels
    c. marveling
    d. marvel

30. a. no change
    b. it was
    c. it has been
    d. its

Use the sentence below to answer questions 31 through 32.
Because of his credulous nature, they took advantage of him and tricked him time and time again.

31. Credulous means:
    a. credibility
    b. gullible
    c. finances
    d. celebrity

32. What is the simple subject of this sentence?
    a. him
    b. nature
    c. they
    d. time

Answer the following item.
33. Which sentence is written correctly?
    a. Due to the time-sensitive nature of the request, the lawyer faxed the document to the judge.
    b. Due to the time-sensitive nature of the request the lawyer faxed the document to the judge.
    c. Due to the time-sensitive nature of the request, the lawyer had faxed the document to the judge.
    d. Due to the time-sensitive nature of the request; the lawyer had faxed the document to the judge.

Read the sentence below and answer questions 34 through 36.
The clerk absconded with the company's payroll.

34. This is a(n) _____ sentence.
    a. imperative
    b. interrogative
    c. exclamatory
    d. declarative

35. What is the simple predicate of this sentence?
    a. absconded with the company's payroll
    b. the clerk
    c. with the company's payroll
    d. absconded

36. Absconded means:
    a. fled.
    b. expired.
    c. invested.
    d. retreated.

Answer the following items.

37. Which of the sentences below is most clear and correct?
    a. The puppies were found by Mr. and Mrs. Gilbert when they were six weeks old.
    b. Mr. and Mrs. Gilbert found the puppies when they were six weeks old.
    c. Mr. and Mrs. Gilbert found the puppies at the age of six weeks.
    d. Six weeks old, Mr. and Mrs. Gilbert found the puppies.

38. The PTA held ___ annual fundraiser.
    a. its
    b. there
    c. their
    d. it's

> **The door swung open.**
> **We spun around.**
> **We saw Kyle Adams.**
> **He staggered into the room.**

39. To improve sentence fluency, how could you state the information above in a single sentence?
    a. When the door swung open and we saw Kyle Adams, he staggered into the room as we spun around.
    b. We saw Kyle Adams as the door swung open and he staggered into the room, as we spun around.
    c. When the door swung open, we spun around and saw Kyle Adams as he staggered into the room.
    d. As he staggered in the room, we saw Kyle Adams and the door swung open; then we spun around.

Read the following medication directions, then answer questions 40 through 44.
Directions: Take at bedtime for abdominal discomfort caused by overindulgence in food or drink. Empty one package in ½ glass of cool water. Drink while effervescing. Dosage may be repeated hourly or as directed by a physician.

40. In which form does this medication come?
    a. powder
    b. liquid
    c. tablet
    d. pill

41. Effervescing means:
    a. melting.
    b. bubbling.
    c. souring.
    d. defrosting.

42. This medication should be taken:
    a. before onset of pain.
    b. at bedtime.
    c. every 30 minutes.
    d. on an empty stomach.

43. Under what circumstances is it permissible to take this medication more frequently than as indicated?
    a. If you eat and drink too much.
    b. If you have more than two packages.
    c. If it doesn't effervesce.
    d. If your doctor tells you to increase it.

44. Once each hour means:
    a. once every 60 minutes.
    b. once on the hour.
    c. once between hours.
    d. approximately one time within the hour.

Answer the following item.
She worked hard to perpetrate the memory of her mother's good deeds.

45. What is the error in this sentence?
    a. mother's
    b. perpetrate
    c. worked
    d. memory

Use the sentence below to answer questions 46 through 47.
The rapacity of our vile, disgusting, and despicable stepfather was not satisfied until he had taken all that we had.

46. Which words are redundant in the sentence above?
    a. rapacity, despicable
    b. rapacity, vile
    c. vile, disgusting
    d. disgusting, despicable

47. Rapacity means:
    a. greed.
    b. dissatisfaction.
    c. reparation.
    d. guilt.

Use this passage to answer questions 48 through 50.
Precautionary Statement: This insect repellent is hazardous to humans. Warning: Harmful if swallowed. May cause eye injury. Do not get into eyes or on lips. To apply to face, spray palm of hand and rub on. Do not apply to excessively sunburned or damaged skin. Use sparingly, with close supervision, on small children. May cause skin reaction in some cases.

48. A precautionary statement:
    a. describes uses of the product.
    b. provides the contents of the product.
    c. lists possible dangers of inappropriate use.
    d. explains how to use the product.

49. Hazardous means:
     a. wasteful.
     b. harmful.
     c. deciduous.
     d. hindering.

50. Use sparingly means to:
     a. apply lavishly.
     b. to massage in thoroughly.
     c. apply moderately.
     d. save some for another time.

Answer the following items.

51. Which sentence is the clearest?
     a. Written by your supervisor, there is a letter in your post office box.
     b. There is a letter written in your post office box by your supervisor.
     c. There is a letter in your post office box written by your supervisor.
     d. By your supervisor, a letter is written in your post office box.

52. Which phrase is misplaced in the sentence below?
     Jennifer mailed a sympathy card to the family of the dead man in a hurry.
     a. in a hurry
     b. to the relatives
     c. Jennifer mailed a sympathy card
     d. of the dead man

Fill-in the blanks in the sentences for questions 53 and 54.

53. Johanna _____ broke the ceramic vase.
     a. on accident
     b. accidently
     c. acidentily
     d. accidentally

54. The veterinarian stood _____ as Tyrone and Misha looked at _____ dog in the cage.
     a. stationery, their
     b. stationary, their
     c. stationery, they're
     d. stationary, they're

Complete the following sentence.

55. Yesterday, Mia
     a. arrives late.
     b. will arrive late.
     c. arrived late.
     d. will have arrived late.

END OF THE TEST

English and Language Usage Practice Test
Answer Key

1.	a	20.	c	39.	c
2.	d	21.	b	40.	a
3.	c	22.	c	41.	b
4.	b	23.	b	42.	b
5.	b	24.	a	43.	d
6.	b	25.	b	44.	a
7.	d	26.	a	45.	b
8.	c	27.	a	46.	c
9.	a	28.	c	47.	a
10.	d	29.	a	48.	c
11.	b	30.	a	49.	b
12.	a	31.	b	50.	c
13.	c	32.	c	51.	c
14.	c	33.	a	52.	a
15.	a	34.	d	53.	d
16.	d	35.	d	54.	b
17.	b	36.	a	55.	c
18.	d	37.	b		
19.	c	38.	a		

Section VI: Comprehensive Examination

DIRECTIONS: The examination you are about to take is multiple-choice with only one correct answer per item. Photocopy the answer sheet on this page to record your choices. Read the questions on the examination carefully and select one correct answer for each test item. When you have completed the practice test, you may check your answers with those listed on the answer key that follows the Comprehensive Examination.

Answer Sheet

1.	a	b	c	d		21.	a	b	c	d
2.	a	b	c	d		22.	a	b	c	d
3.	a	b	c	d		23.	a	b	c	d
4.	a	b	c	d		24.	a	b	c	d
5.	a	b	c	d		25.	a	b	c	d
6.	a	b	c	d		26.	a	b	c	d
7.	a	b	c	d		27.	a	b	c	d
8.	a	b	c	d		28.	a	b	c	d
9.	a	b	c	d		29.	a	b	c	d
10.	a	b	c	d		30.	a	b	c	d
11.	a	b	c	d		31.	a	b	c	d
12.	a	b	c	d		32.	a	b	c	d
13.	a	b	c	d		33.	a	b	c	d
14.	a	b	c	d		34.	a	b	c	d
15.	a	b	c	d		35.	a	b	c	d
16.	a	b	c	d		36.	a	b	c	d
17.	a	b	c	d		37.	a	b	c	d
18.	a	b	c	d		38.	a	b	c	d
19.	a	b	c	d		39.	a	b	c	d
20.	a	b	c	d						

Comprehensive Examination

1. A certain star is 43,056,000 million miles away. What is this number in scientific notation?
   a. 43.056×10^6
   b. 43.056×10^7
   c. 4.3056×10^6
   d. 4.3056×10^7

2. Janine has a recipe that calls for $1^3/_4$ cups of fruit. The recipe serves eight. She plans to prepare the recipe for a group of 20 people. How many cups of fruit will be in the mixture?
   a. $3^1/_2$ cups
   b. $8^3/_4$ cups
   c. $4^3/_8$ cups
   d. $^7/_{10}$ cups

3. Membranes in human cells served to protect the cell by allowing only some substances to pass through. This means that the cells are:
   a. selectively homeostatic.
   b. selectively isotonic.
   c. selectively permeable.
   d. selectively eukaryotic.

4. Find the value of the expression $2xy + 3x - 7y$ when $x = -1$ and $y = 2$.
   a. 7
   b. −21
   c. −7
   d. 21

5. The number of watts in a light bulb is equal to the number of amps times the number of volts times the unit lengths of wire (watts = volts x amps x unit lengths of wire). How would you find the number of amps if you know the number of watts, number of volts and number of unit lengths of wire?
   a. amps = watts x volts x unit lengths of wire

   b. amps = $\dfrac{\text{watts}}{\text{volts x unit lengths of wire}}$

   c. amps = $\dfrac{\text{volts}}{\text{watts x unit lengths of wire}}$

   d. amps = $\dfrac{\text{volts x unit lengths of wire}}{\text{watts}}$

6. A 15% discount is given if a certain bill is paid with cash. Suppose the bill is $50 and the patron pays with cash. What will the patron actually pay?
    a. $42.50
    b. $49.25
    c. $7.50
    d. $0.75

7. An essential step in the production of electrical energy is conduction. <u>Conduct</u> means:
    a. condition.
    b. transfigure.
    c. concur.
    d. transmit.

8. "Ms. Greene reported that last week the street lights have not come on at night." Which of the following statements is written correctly?
    a. Ms. Greene reported last week that the street lights are not coming on at night.
    b. Ms. Greene reported that last week the street lights have not come on at night.
    c. Ms. Greene reported that last week the street lights did not come on at night.
    d. Ms. Greene reported that last week the street lights would not come on at night.

9. The stomach is located in the
    a. dorsal body cavity.
    b. thoracic body cavity.
    c. pelvic body cavity.
    d. abdominal body cavity.

Read the following passage and answer Questions 10 through 15.

Who Runs the Exchanges?

As temples of free enterprise, the world's stock exchanges have traditionally been run by the people who set them up in the first place. They are much like very exclusive private clubs. In many countries, membership can be bought, provided the current members agree to the admission and a vacancy, or "seat," exists. The price is high - up to about $375,000 in New York and a staggering $6.6 million in Tokyo. In other countries, such as Britain, membership is not limited to a fixed number of "seats," but is open to any firm able to meet the entry requirements.

The members make the stock exchange rules, which must conform with the laws of the country. In some countries, an independent body, such as the Securities & Exchange Commission in the United States, has been created to watch over stock exchanges' day-to-day conduct on behalf of the public.

Reader's Digest (1990). The Privileged and Risky World of The Stock Market. *How in the World?* page 38.

---

10. The author's attitude toward the system by which the stock exchange is run is:
    a. humorous.
    b. approving.
    c. matter of fact.
    d. critical.

11. The article could also be titled:
    a. Securities and Exchange Commissions.
    b. The Price of Doing Business.
    c. The Stock Exchange at Home and Abroad.
    d. Stock Exchange Memberships.

12. The author mentions "temples" and "very exclusive private clubs":
    a. so the reader can recognize the extravagance of the system.
    b. to serve as a means to engage the reader.
    c. to express the real reason why the author has taken the time to write this article.
    d. to convey the author's overall distrust of the system.

13. If the maximum cost for membership in the New York Stock Exchange is $375,000 and the maximum cost for membership in the Tokyo Stock Exchange is $6,600,000, the maximum New York membership rate is what percentage of the maximum Tokyo membership rate?
    a. 17.6%.
    b. .06%.
    c. .176%.
    d. 6%.

14. According to this passage, independent agencies are needed in some countries to:
    a. regulate trade between them and Japan.
    b. monitor the daily operations of the stock exchange.
    c. screen the eligibility of candidates for membership.
    d. maintain a more competitive stock market.

15. The price for a vacancy or seat in the New York Stock Exchange:
    a. is substantially higher than in Tokyo.
    b. has increased in recent years.
    c. is substantially lower than in Tokyo.
    d. is 6.6 million dollars.

You are assigned to test the materials in different soil samples. The results are presented in the table below.

Nutrient Filtrate Data Table				
	Soil Sample			
Nutrient	Sample 1	Sample 2		
Nitrates	yes	yes		
Phosphates	yes	no		

16. Which of the following assumptions can be inferred from the existing data?
    a. Different soils contain different nutrients.
    b. Sample 1 is the best soil.
    c. Nitrates are more frequently found in soil than are phosphates.
    d. Most plants thrive in nitrate-rich soil.

17. The class was given an assignment to pour exactly 500 mL of distilled water into a graduated cylinder. Haleh attempted to do this five times. The amounts he poured were 500.9 mL, 499.8 mL, 500.1 mL, 499.7 mL, and 500.1 mL. The results Haleh obtained were:
    a.   precise but not accurate.
    b.   accurate but not precise.
    c.   both accurate and precise.
    d.   neither accurate nor precise.

18. Hydrogen, the lightest known chemical element, is reported to exist as a metallic liquid on the planet Jupiter; whereas on earth it only exists in a gaseous state. It can therefore be deduced that Jupiter, relative to earth, has a significantly:
    a.   lower atmospheric pressure.
    b.   higher surface temperature.
    c.   higher atmospheric pressure.
    d.   lower surface temperature.

19. Which of the following best describes the flow of energy and biomass in an ecosystem?
    a.   Biomass flow is unidirectional and the flow of energy is cyclical.
    b.   Energy flow is unidirectional and biomass flow is cyclical.
    c.   Biomass flow is cyclical and the flow of energy is cyclical.
    d.   Energy flow is unidirectional and biomass flow is unidirectional.

Questions 20 through 24 relate to the graph below.

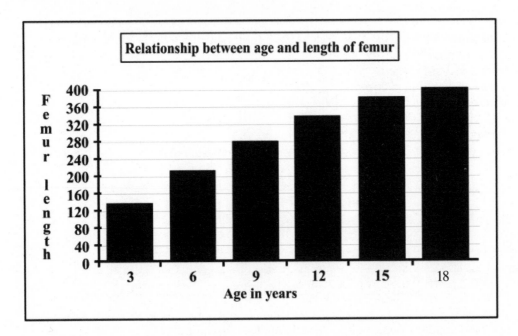

20. Which of the following assumptions can be made from the graph?
    a.   There is an indirect relationship between age and length of femur.
    b.   There is a direct relationship between age and length of femur.
    c.   Age is a constant and length of the femur is a variable.
    d.   Age and length of femur are mutually exclusive.

21. 200 is approximately what percent of the femur growth at age 12?
    a. 82%
    b. 59%
    c. 50%
    d. 21%

22. What is the percentage of increase in the femur length from age 6 to age 18?
    a. 45%
    b. 50%
    c. 82%
    d. 180%

23. What percentage of total femur growth is achieved by age 6 (round to the nearest ten percent)?
    a. 10%
    b. 20%
    c. 40%
    d. 60%

24. The greatest period of femur growth according to the graph is:
    a. 3-6 years.
    b. 6-9 years.
    c. 9-12 years.
    d. 12-15 years.

You have just completed an experiment to measure your lung air capacity. The results are presented in the table below. Tidal air is the air that flows in and out of the lungs when ordinarily breathing. Reserve air is the air that can still be expelled from the lungs after ordinary exhalation. Complemental air is the air that can be inhaled above that normally taken into the lungs.

Lung Capacity	Measurement
Tidal air	27 cubic inches (0.45 liter)
Reserve air	85 cubic inches (1.42 liters)
Complemental air	110 cubic inches (1.83 liters)
Total vital capacity	222 cubic inches (3.70 liters)

25. Looking at the above table, which of the following statements is true?
    a. A person's total vital capacity is dependent on the tidal, reserve, and complemental air.
    b. The amount of air used during normal breathing is greater than the reserve air.
    c. Complemental air has the greatest effect on vital capacity.
    d. Tidal air equals complemental air minus reserve air.

26. Based on data provided in the chart, determine how many cubic inches are in a liter.
    a. 1 liter = 60 cubic inches
    b. 1 liter = 45 cubic inches
    c. 1 liter = .60 cubic inches
    d. 1 liter = 16.6 cubic inches

27. Complemental air may be represented by or likened to a:
    a.   deflated auto tire.
    b.   partially inflated balloon.
    c.   fully expanded accordion bellow.
    d.   collapsed lung.

28. An appropriate synonym for <u>reserve</u> is:
    a.   stored.
    b.   expired.
    c.   residual.
    d.   minimal.

Use the information in the table below to answer question 29.

A class project was to determine the number of gene frequencies in the class. The table below represents the findings.

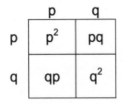

29. Which of the following formulas is appropriate?
    a. $2p^2 + 2pq + q^2 = 100\% = 1$
    b. $2p^2 + q + 2q^2 = 100\% = 1$
    c. $p^2 + pq + 2q^2 = 100\% = 1$
    d. $p^2 + 2pq + q^2 = 100\% = 1$

30. Suppose one parent is heterozygous for a certain trait, while the other parent is homozygous recessive for the same trait. There are two offspring. What are the chances that **both** are homozygous recessive?
    a.   25%
    b.   50%
    c.   75%
    d.   100%

31. If a genetic mutation involves the substitution of one purine base for another in the interior of messenger RNA, known to code for a specific protein, the resulting protein is likely to have:
    a.   several different amino acids from those found in the normal protein.
    b.   one different amino acid in the altered protein.
    c.   two different amino acids in the altered protein.
    d.   no changes in the potentially altered protein.

32. A prescription is written for a certain medication. Typically, the medication costs $1.80 per pill, but with insurance, the price is $1.17 per pill. What is the percent reduction in price per pill?
    a. 65%
    b. 63%
    c. 37%
    d. 35%

33. Directions for a certain medication indicate that the dosage is 15 mg per 25 pounds. The prescription for a person weighing 120 pounds would be how many milligrams?
    a. 200 mg
    b. 72 mg
    c. 16 mg
    d. 12 mg

34. What word most closely describes homeostasis?
    a. instability
    b. movement
    c. rest
    d. stability

35. In which of these ways does the muscular system work with the digestive system?
    a. movement
    b. protection
    c. impulse monitoring
    d. calcium absorption

36. What is the **difference** between a primary and secondary consumer in a food chain?
    a. Secondary consumers are herbivores.
    b. Primary consumers are omnivores.
    c. Primary consumers are herbivores.
    d. Secondary consumers are producers.

37. Which statement is true about epithelial tissue?
    a. It has its own blood supply.
    b. It cannot easily regenerate.
    c. There are three major types.
    d. It serves as a covering.

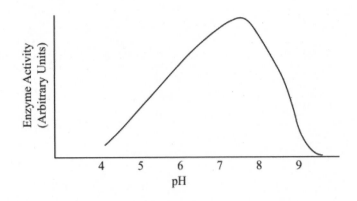

38. Which statement can be made about the graph?
    a.   As pH level increases, enzyme activity increases and then decreases.
    b.   As pH level decreases, enzyme activity increases and then decreases.
    c.   As pH level increases, enzyme activity decreases and then increases.
    d.   As pH level decreases, enzyme activity decreases and then increases.

39. The optimal pH for the enzyme in the graph is approximately:
    a.   9.5.
    b.   4.0.
    c.   7.0.
    d.   7.6.

END OF THE TEST

Answers to Comprehensive Examination

ANSWERS		EXPLANATIONS
1.	d	Recall that a number in scientific notation must be between 1.00 and 9.99. In this case, just move the decimal 7 places to the right.
2.	c	Set up a proportion and solve for x. That is: $\dfrac{1\frac{3}{4}\text{ cups}}{8\text{ servings}} = \dfrac{x\text{ cups}}{20\text{ servings}}$ Change the mixed fraction to an improper fraction. $\dfrac{\frac{7}{4}}{8} = \dfrac{x}{20}$ Cross multiply to get $35 = 8x$ and divide both sides by 8 to get $x = \dfrac{35}{8}$ and simplify to $4\frac{3}{8}$.
3.	c	Recall the definition of "selectively permeable" from the science section.
4.	b	Substitute -1 for x and 2 for y. Then, $2(-1)(2) + 3(-1) - 7(2) = -4 - 3 - 14 = -21$.
5.	b	Watts = amps x volts x unit lengths of wire. Since watts is the product of the other three and the inverse operation of multiplication is division, divide both sides by volts x unit lengths of wire.
6.	a	$50(1 - .15) = 50(.85) = 42.50$ Since the discount is 15%, subtract 15% from 100% and then multiply the difference by 50 OR $50(.15) = \$7.50$, so $50.00 - \$7.50 = \$42.50$. Calculate the discount first, then subtract from the total bill.
7.	d	Synonym for conduct
8.	c	Since this happened last week, the verb tense must reflect that.
9.	d	Recall the cavities in the human body from the Science section.
10.	d	Note the second sentence and words such as "staggering" in the text.
11.	d	Think about the overall picture provided by the text.
12.	d	Read these words in context to get an overall idea.
13.	d	$375,000 / 6,600,000 = 375 / 6,600 = .06 \times 100\% = 6\%$
14.	b	Refer to the text.
15.	c	Refer to the text.

16.	a	The other possibilities do not reflect the basic information presented in the table.
17.	c	He poured multiple measures and each was quite close to the desired 500 mL.
18.	c	Since hydrogen appears as a liquid on Jupiter, there must be higher pressure condensing the elements and molecules.
19.	b	Recall that mass is neither created nor destroyed. It just changes forms. Energy flows from a high level to a lower level.
20.	b	Based on the graph, as age increases, so does femur length.
21.	b	Divide 200 by 340 and you get .588 or 59%.
22.	c	$\dfrac{400-220}{220} = .818$ or 82% To find the percent increase, subtract the beginning amount from the ending amount and divide by the beginning amount.
23.	d	$\dfrac{220}{400} \approx .55$ Of the final length, how much is achieved by age 6? Divide the length at age 6 by the final length.
24.	a	Find the differences between adjacent bars and decide which has the highest difference.
25.	a	The total air capacity is found by adding the three types of air.
26.	a	Set up a proportion. $\dfrac{27\,\text{cubic inches}}{.45\,\text{liters}} = \dfrac{x\,\text{cubic inches}}{1.0\,\text{liters}}$ Cross multiply to get $.45x = 27$ and divide both sides by .45.
27.	c	Check the definition of complemental air, and think about how else this could be represented.
28.	a	"Stored" is a synonym for "reserve."
29.	d	$p^2 + pq + qp + q^2 = p^2 + 2pq + q^2$
30.	a	Draw a Punnett square with one parent Aa and the other parent aa. Determine the cross. You should notice that there is a 50% chance of an offspring being homozygous recessive. This is the case for every offspring. So, multiply .5 by .5 to get 25%.
31.	b	Since only one purine base has been altered, only one amino acid can be different.
32.	d	Subtract the discounted price from the original price and divide by the original price. $\dfrac{1.80-1.17}{1.80} = 35\%$
33.	b	Set up a proportion and solve. $\dfrac{15\,\text{mg}}{25\,\text{lbs}} = \dfrac{x\,\text{mg}}{120\,\text{lbs}}$ and cross multiply to get $25x = 15(120)$ and divide both sides by 25.

34.	d	Recall the definition from the Science section.
35.	a	Smooth muscle aids in movement of food through digestive system.
36.	c	Review the food chain from the Science section.
37.	d	Review the tissue discussion from the Science section.
38.	a	As pH goes from 4 to about 7.9, the enzyme activity increases. From 7.9 to about 9.5, the enzyme activity decreases.
39.	d	Find the peak. This is, by definition, the highest level of activity.

CONGRATULATIONS! This preparation guide has provided you with information about specific content areas and tips for taking the Test of Essential Academic Skills. Use your score on the Comprehensive Examination to determine what to do next. If you need more practice, review the study guide's explanations to expand your understanding in areas where you might need remediation.

If you would like additional TEAS preparatory material, a 100-item, on-line practice examination is also available. The examination is designed to reflect the TEAS™ in content, format, and style. In order to maximize the learning experience, students are provided with explanations for all correct and incorrect responses chosen. For more information, please visit www.atitesting.com.